ACTIVE YEARS FOR YOUR AGING DOG

ACTIVE YEARS FOR YOUR AGING DOG

Bernard S. Hershhorn, D.V.M.

HAWTHORN BOOKS, INC.
Publishers / New York
A Howard & Wyndham Company

ACTIVE YEARS FOR YOUR AGING DOG

Library of Congress Catalog Card Number: 78-52966

ISBN: 0-8015-4599-4

1 2 3 4 5 6 7 8 9 10

To Ida and Max Hershhorn—
my beloved departed mother and father—
Jewish parents who never said
"You must grow up to be a doctor or a lawyer,"
but instead only
"Be whatever will make you happiest, but always be a *mensch*."

Contents

PART ONE

YOU AND YOUR AGING DOG

Preface

The nature of dog ownership and dog owners has undergone many changes during the hundred-odd years that veterinary medicine has been a recognized profession in this country. From the animal that had to fend for itself and was rarely tolerated inside the house, the dog has become an integral part of the family. Even farm and other working dogs share much more of the lives of their human families. This change in canine-human interaction has progressively been producing a new kind of dog owner. It used to be a client would drop off his dog saying, "He doesn't feel good, doc. Check him over, fix him up, and send me the bill." He didn't particularly care what was wrong with his dog as long as the doctor "fixed him up." Increasingly larger numbers of dog owners now not only take an active interest in their dog's illness but want to know about, and understand, the disorder. They want to feel that they are sharing in the diagnostic and therapeutic processes which will help their dog to get well.

The days are gone when a client would accept a veterinarian's superficial instructions of "just give him these pills for a few days and he'll be fine." You want to know exactly what is wrong. You want to understand the details of what is ailing your aging dog: and you don't want to be left "out in the dark" or confused by a maze of medical jargon. *You want to be taken into your doctor's medical confidence!* This book was written to do just that and to serve as a guide to preventive medicine as well as to the problems that you, your dog, and your family veterinarian may have to cope with at various times as your dog ages. Most importantly, it was written to advise you on what you personally can do to help both your dog and your veterinarian in dealing with age-related health questions.

This is *not* a text on the diagnosis and treatment of canine illnesses and should *never* be used as such. To do so could seriously jeopardize the health and very life of your dog. Your family veterinarian is the trained and qualified medical professional to properly care for your dog. By using this book as intended, however, you can, in a case of illness, assist your veterinarian to arrive at a diagnosis and institute therapy much sooner, thereby helping to prolong your dog's life.

Who is this book for? It is for *you,* the owner of—

- an aged dog, in good or in poor health. This book will help you to understand what may happen or has already happened to your dog and what you can do to help.

- a middle-aged dog. You will be made aware of the many things you can do preventively to increase the chances of your dog reaching old age in good health and staying that way much longer.

- a young dog. You have an entire dog lifetime to use the concepts presented here to improve your young one's chances of lifelong good health and a happy old age.

If you have a mature dog in good health, read "Aging and Staying Young" followed by "When Your Dog Is Sick." Then read the rest of the book as your interests direct.

If your mature dog is already ill, read about the particular problem in "Specific Diseases or Disorders," followed directly by "When Your Dog Is Sick" and then "Aging and Staying Young." The rest of the book can be read while your dog is recovering.

If you have a middle-aged or young dog, read the book in the order presented, although you might wish to leave ''Specific Diseases or Disorders'' for last. Read it through leisurely and then review ''Aging and Staying Young'' as well as ''When Your Dog Is Sick.''

If you still have unanswered questions about the aging canine, or anything else pertaining to your dog's health, consult your family veterinarian. He or she is truly your dog's best friend—*after you, of course!*

This book should help you understand—

- the aging process.
- how to help your dog better to deal with aging.
- how to know when your dog is ill.

It will—

- tell you how to help your veterinarian help your dog.
- provide information about many specific diseases or disorders of old age.
- tell you what to do in certain emergencies.
- help you to understand how you and your dog *together* can face the inevitable when time does at last run out.

If I have succeeded in doing these things for you and your dog, my purpose in writing this book will have been achieved and my efforts will have been well spent.

The use of brand names or manufacturers' names in the text does not in any way imply an endorsement of those products or manufacturers by either the author or the publisher except where specifically so stated.

Acknowledgments

From its inception and throughout the writing of this book, there have been a number of people who have helped me in various ways.

To B. P., whose patience and understanding made it all possible, and to Effie Cooper, who introduced me to my publisher, my thanks.

To Robert Oskam of Hawthorn Books, who recognized the need for this book and asked me to write it, my thanks for his confidence, support, and constructive editing.

Anne and Milton Hershhorn, Joan Schiffer, Cindy Laird, and Irene Soskin either read portions of the manuscript, offering helpful criticism, or otherwise made very valuable suggestions. I am grateful for their assistance and especially for their faith in me during my not infrequent moments of doubt.

To the firms who kindly permitted the use of their material in some of the tables and illustrations, I offer my appreciation.

My gratitude to the late John Vogel, kennelman *extraordinaire,* who taught me during my early years of practice about the nonmedical individual needs of all hospitalized dogs and, in particular, the very special needs of such aged dogs. I owe him much.

And thank you to all my geriatric patients—including Loki, Tinker Belle, Hank, Liebchen, Michael, Genghis, Gypsy, Krismus, Jezebel, Maggie, Tommy, Princess, Ginger, Brutus, Shadow, Winston, Muffin, Pooh, Giotto, and Cleo—and their owners, all of whom loved their dogs, helped me to help them, and actively shared with me the responsibilities of prolonging an active and happy life for their pets.

Introduction

Age does not depend upon years, but upon temperament and health. Some . . . are born old, and some never grow so.

—Tryon Edwards

James A. Garfield, twentieth president of the United States, once said, "If wrinkles must be written upon our brows, let them not be written upon the heart. The spirit should never grow old." When is a dog considered to be aging? When is he to be called old? It really depends on the breed of dog and on whether you are talking about physiological age or chronological age, as these two don't necessarily coincide. A dog of fourteen may be old by his numerical years but his body systems may well be functioning as normally as those of a much younger canine. Should he be called old? The dog of seven who has been chronically ill, whose body systems can just barely sustain him, who looks and acts worn out—should he be called young? All of us know people who are old "before their time" at fifty and others who, at eighty or ninety, are still physically active and belie their chronological age. "Old" must always be qualified in relation to physiological or chronological age. It must also carry with it a qualification based on breed or type of dog. Many giant breeds are physiologically old by their eighth or ninth birthday, while schnauzers, spaniels, terriers, and others often reach fourteen and fifteen in a biologically sound state that belies their years.

As of this writing, no one knows for sure exactly what causes the changes observed in the aging process. Nor do we know how to stop or permanently reverse them. There is no Fountain of Youth—yet! But we are able to recognize most of these changes, often early enough to do something about them. The rate of development of many can be slowed down, and a few of these changes can actually be reversed, if only for short periods of time. In an increasingly large number of cases, treatment is available to alleviate, if not cure, the problems which do develop. Let me hasten to add, however, that any given aging dog is certainly not going to develop all, or even most, of the problems covered in this book, although he will likely have one or another from time to time as he grows older.

Who then is the aging canine, and who the old? From seven years on almost all dogs can be considered to be aging, and the dog who is chronologically *or* physiologically fourteen or more can surely be called old. But old doesn't necessarily mean falling apart at the seams or ready to pass out of the picture. As I have tried to make clear in this book, many such old dogs can continue to live happy and meaningful lives for another two, three, five, or more years.

When I started in practice as a doctor of veterinary medicine in 1955, one seldom saw a dog who was more than ten years old. The *average* life span for all canine breeds has been increased by fifty percent or more over the past thirty years, and dogs are living much longer today than ever before.

If you acquire a new puppy today of any breed, except the giant ones, immunize it effectively and regularly, feed and exercise it properly, and do what is necessary to maintain it in good health; you can reasonably expect it to live to be fifteen, or even eighteen or twenty years of age. Back in the fifties, that span would have been about twelve years and before World War II substantially less.

One of the major factors in increasing the longevity of dogs has been the conquest and continuing control of three major infectious diseases—canine distemper, canine infectious hepatitis, and leptospirosis. Dog owners have also become more knowledgeable, more concerned, and more willing to learn about their pet's health problem and so are able to give better care. Canine foods and feeding concepts have improved enormously during this time. Your dog is now far more likely to be fed a properly balanced diet than before, when the old "feed him table scraps and throw him a bone" diet used to constitute canine "nutrition."

The science and art of veterinary medicine has also advanced, almost by geometric progression, with the result that your family veterinarian today is able to diagnose and successfully treat numerous conditions, particularly those of geriatric dogs, that thirty years ago were "treated" by euthanasia.

Almost all dog owners are consciously or subconsciously deeply concerned about their dog "getting old," as well as about the problems for dog and owner which can arise from it. We all *know* that aging is inevitable, but we do not have to accept meekly the inevitability, sit back and "become old." There are things which you can do to alter to some degree the problems and timetable of aging. Again, don't misunderstand me! I am not saying that if you provide the absolute best of care for your dog—diet, exercise, veterinary medical care and treatment, love—that he will not have aging problems. I do say that some of those problems can be prevented, others alleviated, and a few learned to live with. The prospect of your dog's aging does not have to be disquieting or fearful. A dog can age gracefully and in reasonable comfort. Your *aged* dog does not have to be an *old* dog.

Western society has tended to relegate its aged members to the background, to a state of being undesirable, unfit, asocial, and just generally, in the way. In the United States especially, there is, and has been for many generations, a youth-oriented culture. To be old is to be ignored! Most Americans do not like to think of themselves as being old or becoming old. So instead of just one word—old—our vocabulary has acquired many euphemisms to substitute for it, such as golden-ager, mature, senior citizen, and others.

Over the past decade, however, this country has undergone a slow change of heart and is beginning to realize the importance of old people and the concern and rights to which they are entitled. Somewhat more slowly, the same realizations are being reached by the owners of aging dogs. They are losing the former concepts that a dog gets old by herself and, when she gets ''seriously'' sick, should be gotten rid of because ''she's no good anymore.''

Your own attitude toward growing old will surely be reflected in your dog's aging. People do not always have to give in to the aging process without a fight. They can and should—but all too often don't—take simple preventive actions throughout their lives to better equip themselves to deal with the supposed ''ravages of age''. Through your considerate and considered thought and action, your dog can do likewise!

PART ONE

You and Your Aging Dog

1
Aging and Staying Young

What is old age? What is aging? Why do we age? Why does one begin to age more rapidly than another? Why are some only "as old as they feel" while others are as old or older than they look?

Throughout human history, there have been endless numbers of theories postulated in an attempt to answer these questions about the aging process. Currently, there are three which have received some degree of widespread acceptance. That is, until newer ones replace them. With all our advances in science and technology, no one yet truly understands why we age.

The first theory states that cells of the body undergo mutation with the passage of time, and these mutated cells are less able to perform their functions than normal cells. Another theory declares that each body cell has a finite amount of essential enzymes which eventually becomes exhausted so that the cell "wears out." The third theory claims that harmful products accumulate within the cells and tissues which increasingly interfere with the cells' normal functions. Each theory has its active proponents and vocal opponents, which is as it should be in all scientific investigation. Perhaps one is correct or all three or none. For the present, we simply do not know for sure.

Life Span

It has been said that, like a clock, life ticks away with every beat of the heart. There is probably a good deal more scientific truth in that statement than its unknown author intended or was aware of. There is a definite relationship between the size of an animal's body and both its heart and respiratory rates. Larger species of mammals, like whales, tick away more slowly than smaller ones such as dogs. The former have a slower metabolic rate, breathe much slower, and their hearts beat less frequently than dogs. Different sizes of mammalian species seem to live for the same *relative* length of biological time, when measured against their own individual internal clocks.

Regardless of this supposedly relative uniformity of life span among all mammals and a more or less consistent rate of aging, there are factors related to breed and individual idiosyncracy which can significantly lengthen, but more often shorten, a dog's life. The high prevalence of osteosarcoma, a highly malignant type of bone cancer, in the Great Dane drastically shortens the life expectancy of most individuals of that breed. It is quite unusual even today to see a Great Dane older than nine or ten years. Most of the very large and giant breeds, as a group, have an abnormally high rate of idiopathic congestive cardiomyopathy, a serious primary disease of the heart muscle. It is found most often in the St. Bernard, Great Dane, Irish wolfhound, and German shepherd, and with less frequency in many other breeds. It, too, reduces life expectancy.

Mastocytoma, a tumor of the skin, occurs with about twice the frequency in boxers, Labrador retrievers, and Boston terriers as can be expected for other breeds. The incidence in Chihuahuas is close to one-sixth the expected normal. In a somewhat different manner, sex also has an effect on longevity. The frequent occurrence of mammary tumors in the female, as opposed to the less frequent development of tumors of the testicles in males, can shorten the life expectancy of your female canine. The greater incidence of urethral calculi (stones) in males can in a like manner diminish male life expectancy. For a fuller discussion of these breed and sex influences, refer to the individual disorder descriptions in Part Two of this book.

When physiological aging begins, there are certain physical changes in the body. There is a consistent timetable which determines when these changes will take place, at what speed they will proceed, or how much damage any of them will do. Siblings, even twins, may show tremendous variation. Each organ and system of the living body is composed of millions of cells. Beyond a certain undetermined point in life, dying cells are not replaced rapidly enough or at all. Thus almost all organs and systems of the aging dog become less capable of performing their vital functions. In muscles, this results in decreased size and strength. In the kidneys, their ability to selectively separate beneficial from harmful substances in the blood and urine diminishes. In nerve tissue, the ability to transmit impulses, as well as the speed of such transmission, is decreased.

Fortunately, the living body has a substantial reserve built into most of its components. Hence the aged dog can live quite satisfactorily as long as those component organs and systems can meet the *minimum* level of function compatible with supporting normal life. However, variation from that normal life pattern of any given aged dog may render some or all of the components inadequate to sustain life. Geriatric dogs are less capable of adapting to internal or external changes, have a reduced organ function reserve, and are generally impaired to some degree in their body's ability to heal sick or injured tissues.

Until science finds a way to change it, aging remains a normal part of life. But it brings about a decreasing resistance to the wide spectrum of internal and external events that can occasion death. Age itself does not cause death, but the physiological alterations produced by advancing age make death more likely to occur from these many causes.

Three terms relating to length of life are often used interchangeably, when they do, in fact, have different meanings. So let's clarify just what we are talking about.

• Life span—this is the greatest length of life regarded as biologically possible for a given animal or species. It remains the same throughout life.

• Life expectancy—this refers to the probable further length of life of an animal at any given time during that life and varies with age, sex, physical condition, and other factors. At birth it is the same as life span but from that moment on changes throughout the animal's life.

• Longevity—great age or great length of life.

There have been many claims of extreme canine longevity, but few have been accurately documented. Many owners, especially of older dogs, don't seem to be able to remember the exact birthday or even the exact year of their dog's birth. Do you know precisely when your dog was born? A client recently tried to remember—"Well, let me see. We had Duke when I got married and that was six years ago, and I think I was just out of high school when we bought him. Or was it during my senior year? . . . Wait, I know! We got Duke the year my brother broke his leg! . . . But I can't remember which year that was!" Of course, all pedigreed dogs arrive with "papers" showing their birth date, but over the years such papers have a way of disappearing and the determination of age again depends on the owner's memory.

One generally accepted longevity record was set in England by a dog who died in 1963 at the reputed age of twenty-seven and one-quarter years, having spent his entire life with only one owner. That would make the dog equivalent to one hundred forty-two human years by present calculations or one hundred ninety-one by the old seven-to-one ratio!

In my personal experience, the oldest dog I've known was a Manchester terrier who lived with the widow of a well-known song and musical show writer. This dowager canine was at least twenty-one by provable records and could have been another three or four years older, because she had been acquired as an adult. She was in rather good health for her age—cataracts and a somewhat stiff gait, but otherwise reasonably active, in no discomfort, and quite enjoying life. During her twenty-first year, however, she developed a life-threatening uterine infection (pyometra) which required a complete ovariohysterectomy, a serious operation under such conditions of infection. Nevertheless, she came through the surgery and anesthesia with flying colors, continued to live a happy life for almost eight months longer, and then peacefully died in her sleep one night.

Comparative Age

One of the commonest nonmedical questions I am asked by clients is how old their dog is compared to human years. Over the many centuries that the human race has shared its various dwellings with dogs, I know of no definitive work done to compare periods of human and canine life. Through the time in the early fifties when I was a student at veterinary college, the prevailing consensus was that one year of a dog's life was equivalent to seven years of human life. Thus a one-year-old dog was comparable to a seven-year-old child, one of seven to a forty-nine-year-old adult, and a canine of slightly over fourteen to a human centenarian. In

Old at twelve years

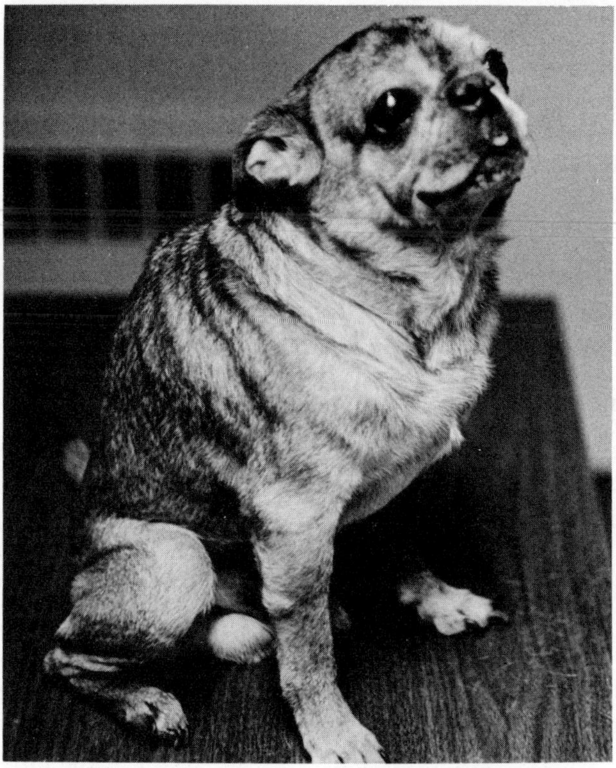

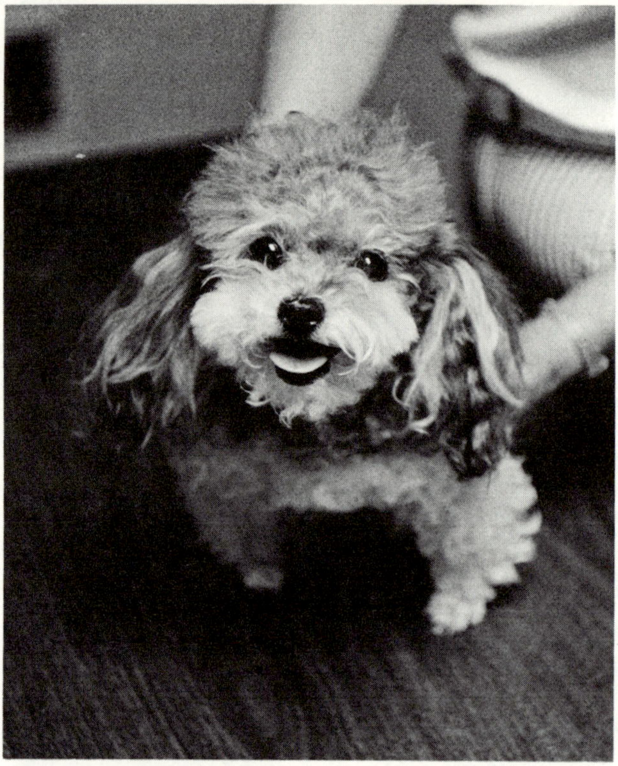

Young at eleven years

most dogs, however, this equation is not borne out by fact. A dog of one year is far more physically and emotionally developed than a child of seven. While the dog may yet retain some puppyish traits, it generally behaves much like a young adult. A ten-year-old canine rarely has the physical or emotional problems or attitudes of a human septuagenarian. If a dog's years are equivalent to one hundred by the time it is fourteen plus, the many dogs who live to be sixteen or twenty must be considered truly ancient!

During the course of the past two decades, as more attention and research has been directed at geriatrics in both people and canines, a somewhat more probable comparison has been suggested. It acknowledges that puppies and young dogs mature more rapidly during their first two years of life. From then on it equates at a steady rate of one dog year to four human years. It also acknowledges the fact that dogs are living longer lives than they did three and four decades ago.

Canine	*Human*
3 months	5 years
6 months	10 years
1 year	15 years
2 years	24 years
3 years	28 years
4 years	32 years
5 years	36 years
6 years	40 years
7 years	44 years
8 years	48 years
9 years	52 years
10 years	56 years
12 years	64 years
14 years	72 years
16 years	80 years
18 years	88 years
20 years	96 years
21 years	100 years

Yet this comparison still has shortcomings. Beyond approximately fifteen years of age, dogs seem once again to age at a slightly more rapid rate, all other factors being equal. I would like to suggest that after such an age is attained, one canine year is more probably equivalent to five human years. Thus your senior citizen dog would be

16 years	81 years
18 years	91 years
20 years	101 years
21 years	106 years

All these comparative ages, you must bear in mind, are for the "average" dog who is between perhaps ten and seventy pounds and of traditional canine conformation. It is less readily applicable to the giant and toy breeds, and those breeds whose body conformation has been radically altered by selective breeding, such as the English bulldog.

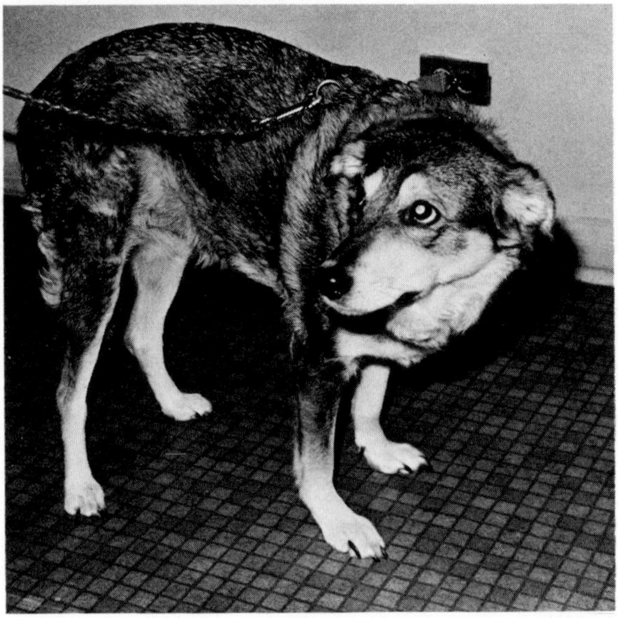

Old at fourteen years. Note the stiff stance of the back legs, the sagging front paws, and the arched back.

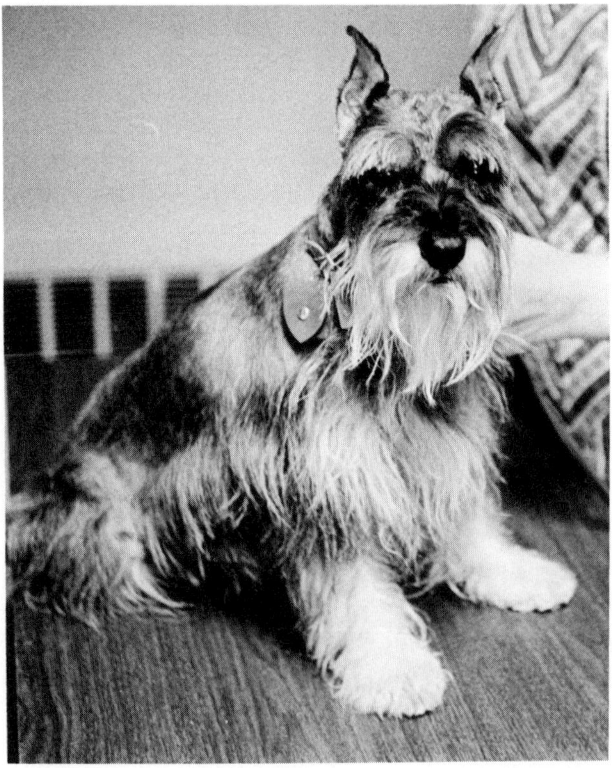

Young at fourteen years. Despite the sleepy appearance caused by his long eyebrows, this dog is alert. Note the erect ears.

Normal Changes as Your Dog Ages

Although the process of aging begins immediately after birth, one cannot reasonably expect to detect such very subtle changes for quite some time and in most dogs not for several years. By the time your dog gets to be five, six, or seven years old, some of these changes can be observed. Many of the earliest signs are often detectable only by a careful physical and laboratory examination. Hence the desirability of having your family veterinarian give your dog an annual geriatric examination starting at about this age. More about this examination later.

Please bear in mind that the changes described here are almost always a normal and expected part of aging but do not necessarily occur in every older dog nor in the particular order set forth here. While they should be looked upon as part of the expected aging process and as nothing to be distressed by, they should not be summarily relegated to the "I don't have to be concerned about them" status. Some of these early normal aging signs can, and do, progress to the point of causing illness. The degree of normality varies, and what is normal for someone else's dog may indeed be normal for yours.

ACTIVENESS

Among the first changes you will notice is a general slowing down in activity. Duke, your energetic friend who is always jumping onto everything and is forever underfoot, doesn't seem to jump as much or with the same vigor. You no longer find yourself tripping over him, and now you can open the refrigerator door without him racing in from wherever he might be. He's not as curious about things around him and is less interested in or disturbed by the activities going on in his environment.

APPETITE

Duke's interest in eating may also be on the wane somewhat, and he is probably eating more slowly. He should not be indulged with special foods or treats, which will make him finicky. Continue to offer him his regular diet unless advised otherwise by your veterinarian. Warming the food will increase its aroma and palatability, thereby providing a greater stimulus to what could be some loss in Duke's sense of smell or taste. You should, of course, check his teeth and gums to be sure that problems in the mouth are not the true source of any changes in eating habits.

TEMPERATURE SENSITIVITY

During the colder time of year, you notice Duke doesn't want to be outside as much as he used to, especially if it is damp. If he is an outdoor dog, you will want to provide warmer bedding and shelter, taking particular care to keep out drafts and moisture. In hot weather, he will probably not run as fast or as far and will seek out shady spots and cooler areas considerably more often than you recall his having done before. He may do more panting or just open-mouth breathing, especially when the humidity is high. You will remember how those long hot summers with temperatures in the 80s and 90sF (27° to 37°C) never seemed to bother him, but now he's showing some discomfort at 75°F (24°C). You can help by limiting his outdoor activities to sunshine hours during the cold, and the early morning or late evening during the heat.

ATTENTIVENESS

One sign of aging which can be very upsetting if you don't fully appreciate what is truly happening, is an increasing inattentiveness and apparent loss of obedience training. When you call to him, Duke seems to be ignoring you, or else he responds so slowly that you are tempted to punish him for disobedience. Nothing of the sort should be done! Duke is, more likely than not, developing a gradual hearing loss. Both the loudness and the range of sounds are being reduced and account for what seems to be inattentiveness. These same changes, plus slight alterations in the nerve pathways leading to, through, and from the brain, account for his noticeably slower response once he does finally pay attention to you. To punish him, or to subject him to obedience retraining, would be a cruel thing which could easily break his spirit and build a wall of distrust and fear between the two of you.

It is quite easy to conduct an objective test of Duke's hearing yourself. Be sure the room is quiet and there are no distracting sounds, lights, or physical vibrations. While he is resting quietly but awake, stand about five feet behind him, being sure he cannot see you. Loudly clap your hands together as you watch his head and ears. If his ears perk up and he turns to see where the sound is coming from, he can still hear quite well. If there is little or no response, there is hearing impairment to some degree. You should then try the same test a bit closer, again being sure that he neither sees you nor feels the vibrations or air currents created by the movement of your hands. Assuming he does respond adequately, you may try again with not so loud a clap or by snapping your fingers, progressively decreasing the volume of the sounds. One caution—do not do these tests in rapid succession, as louder sounds may temporarily diminish response to succeeding quieter ones. Allow at least fifteen to thirty seconds to elapse between each decreased degree of sound.

By means of such testing, you can establish the approximate level of Duke's hearing ability as well as monitor it periodically to detect any further hearing deficiency. Keep in mind, however, that there can be a considerable variation in his ability to hear *spoken* sounds of differing pitch. Therefore his response may be quite different, depending on whether the speaker is a woman or man, child or adult.

SLEEP PATTERNS

When Duke was a very young puppy his twenty-four-hour day was divided into brief repeated cycles of eating, sleeping, and playing which he would try to continue through the night, often resulting in loss of sleep for you. As he matured he was able to follow your patterns and sleep more or less through the night. Older dogs frequently tend to regress toward the earlier multi-cyclic type of sleeping. You may now find Duke napping several times during the day—even when you are home—and perhaps spending a significant portion of the night wide-awake. As with the puppy, feeding him later in the evening will help him to sleep through the night.

ADAPTABILITY

It is not uncommon to find the older dog less adaptable to changes in diet, routine, or environment. Duke always loved riding in the car, bounding about with a *joie de vivre.* He never missed a thing that passed by; now he prefers to lie quietly on the seat snuggled up against you or else on the floor. He may even get an occasional upset stomach and throw up while riding. And he steps in and out of the car with considerably greater care!

In the past it never seemed to bother him if you occasionally got home late for his supper. He'd jovially greet you at the door with little more than a "Hey, what's up?" and race you for the food dish. Now you find that he has thrown up small amounts of yellowish-green stomach fluid due to the increased acidity of a stomach which contains no food. Leaving a small amount of dry food when you go out may solve this upset. Speaking of stomach upset, whenever you had parties, Duke always joined in the fun and most of the time survived the party foods given him by your well-meaning guests. Now he shows less interest in the goings-on, preferring to be by himself in a quieter part of the house. If he does indulge in any party food, he almost always has some digestive disturbance.

COAT AND SKIN

Aging can bring with it many visible physical alterations. The hair around the muzzle will start to show some graying, and the coat will lose much of its former luster, regardless of how effectively you are grooming your dog. The hairs will also become drier and begin to thin out, even to the point of balding in some dogs. You may see small firm pimples or wart-like growths on the skin almost anywhere on the body. These are usually sebaceous gland adenomas, *benign* tumors of the skin's oil glands, which are losing much of their function. If these do not bother Duke, and he does not bother them, it is rarely necessary that anything be done except to carefully avoid scratching them during his daily grooming.

GAIT

Perhaps the surest sign of aging is the development of a stiff, stilted gait even when walking on level ground. This is most likely the result of early osteoarthritis, reduced muscle mass and strength, and some demineralization of bone. After he has been sleeping or lying down for awhile, Duke may get up very slowly and take several minutes of slow stretching before being able to walk with ease. You can help him by providing a warm, soft surface to lie on and, under the supervision of your veterinarian, by administering prescribed physiotherapy.

One morning you may be startled by his not lifting his leg to urinate. Instead he just stands there in a sawhorse stance or, even more startling, squats like a female. Don't worry about his losing his "masculinity" or that he is going through a male menopause! His osteoarthritis is just a little too annoying that day for him to be able to balance himself on three legs.

Duke's toenails may appear to be growing faster than ever before, whereas they are only being worn down less because of his decreased walking and running. You will therefore have to cut or file them more frequently.

MUSCLE TONE

You may observe Duke's abdomen beginning to sag a bit, whether or not he is obese, as the abdominal muscles lose their tone and strength. The female dog who has had puppies may, in addition to a sagging belly, have drooping breasts in her later years. Unless obesity or some of the hormone-related disorders are present, these sagging seniors can be considered to be aging normally and sometimes can have their waistlines trimmed by judicious exercise.

TOILET FUNCTIONS

Over a period of months or years you will notice, if you are a keen observer, a gradual increase in the amount and frequency of urination as well as an increase in the amount of water he is drinking. This is less likely to be diabetes than Duke's physiological adjustment to his slow loss of kidney function efficiency. He may have to be let out more frequently if he isn't paper trained. However, it is vital to his health that you continue to allow him free access to fresh drinking water!

The digestive system is not neglected by aging either. As the secretion of gastric and other digestive juices, as well as the movement of the intestines, become sluggish, there is likely to be less frequent bowel activity which will result in some degree of constipation or flatulence or both.

EYESIGHT

The development of a grayish or bluish haze *inside* the eyes is a normal occurrence and, although it involves the lens of the eye, should not be confused with cataracts. This is not cataract formation, but rather nuclear sclerosis (central hardening) of the lens, a normal aging process. It rarely interferes with vision, although you might notice some reduction in visual acuity under poor light conditions. You can test Duke's general ability to see by yourself. Using a Ping Pong ball and working in a well-lit room, bounce the ball and watch his reaction. When the ball hits the floor he may turn toward it because he heard it bounce, but if he *follows* its movement with his head or eyes, he can see quite well.

SMELL AND TASTE

It is not known with certainty that the senses of smell and taste really decline with advancing age. Certainly many dogs become reluctant to eat the foods that they have been on for most of their years. On the opposite side of the coin, however, we all know at least a dog or two who can sniff out a tasty morsel, no matter how old he gets!

As stated previously, some of the changes normally associated with aging can become progressive and eventually result in illness or disability. We do know with considerable certainty that increasing age brings with it lowered resistance to disease and a longer period of healing and recuperation from even relatively minor illnesses. Specific diseases or disorders are discussed in Part Two of this book.

How to Keep from Becoming "Old"

EXERCISE

Over the past decade, Americans have been swept up in a physical fitness and exercise frenzy which has started an improvement in the overall health of this nation. Jogging, cycling, physical fitness classes, swimming, and similar activities have become topics of everyday discussion with friends and neighbors over dinner and during coffee breaks. For some reason which eludes me, these same fitness-oriented people often do not realize that their aging dog also needs exercise to remain fit and trim. Now please don't rush off and register Duke in the local YMCA. He doesn't need that kind or degree of physical activity—but physical activity he definitely needs!

The amount and type of exercise will of course vary with Duke's physical size and with the state of health of his cardiovascular and musculoskeletal systems, but chronological age in itself is *not* a limiting factor. Snorter, a terrier mix, is far more active at sixteen than Chip, a springer spaniel, is at twelve. Most toy breeds can provide their own necessary exercise, even in an apartment. As a group, they tend to be hyperactive and rarely need to be encouraged to move about unless you've allowed them to become fat. Teaching them to retrieve a thrown object such as a rawhide toy, and playing this game with them for two or three five-minute periods each day will provide the necessary exercise activity.

The medium-size dogs, from miniature schnauzers to retrievers, should have three brisk (for you) walks every day for at least fifteen minutes each, in addition to a five-minute slow trot or toy retrieval game. The larger breeds will require the same brisk walks, but you should add a five-minute run at the end of each walk or have separate running periods. If yours is basically an outdoor dog, you will have to observe him carefully to be certain he is exercising adequately and not just snoozing all day in the backwoods.

I can't imagine anyone in this day and age not knowing the benefits of regular exercise, but just in case . . . ! Properly regulated, exercise can make your dog feel better, look better, perform better, and *probably* live somewhat longer. It will improve normal heart and lung function and reserve, strengthen muscles, keep aging joints flexible, and make him better able to enjoy comfortably his senior years.

Obviously a dog who has developed heart disease, arthritis, or some of the other disorders that sometimes accompany aging, should not be subjected to a program of such activity. But don't get the notion that he needs only peace and quiet, and no exercise at all. With very few exceptions, even such dogs should have *regular* exercise, albeit very limited, and perhaps of a less active or even a passive type. Limbs stiff from joint disease and muscles weakened by the shrinkage of age can both benefit from passive exercise and physiotherapy. Allow your dog to lie on his side or back, whichever is more comfortable for him, and *slowly* flex and extend each leg for several minutes. The muscles and joints are thereby gently exercised, as is the circulatory system.

A word of caution! Before you start any kind of exercise program for an older dog or for one who has a cardiovascular, skeletal, muscular, or kidney disorder, a complete physical examination is in order. Your veterinarian will then be able to knowledgeably advise you on which type, and how much, exercise will be both beneficial and safe for your dog.

Normal play activities should continue throughout life, unless contraindicated for medical reasons, excepting the more strenuous games. Certainly any activity which requires your dog to suddenly stop short or twist and change direction while running should be discontinued. This type of motion readily causes dislocations and joint ligament injuries. The weakening muscles and supporting joint ligaments may no longer have the strength to hold the joint stable against such sudden force applied to it.

Breeds which are predisposed to the intervertebral disc syndrome or "slipped disc"—dachshunds, cocker spaniels, miniature poodles—should not be allowed or encouraged to walk erect on their hind legs or jump up and down on them, either in play or to beg for tidbits, no matter how "cute" it may seem. Although there is as yet no hard evidence to prove it, there is ample circumstantial data to indicate that such jumping or walking exerts tremendous abnormal pressures on the discs and may actually be a cause of certain types of disc protrusion.

The same restrictions apply to any dog who has acquired luxating patellae—slipping of the knee caps, or "trick" knees—or who was born with this structural defect, as is common in so many of the toy breeds. These knee caps slip "out of joint" often enough with just normal walking or running, preventing the leg from bearing weight and causing the dog to hold it up and hop around on three legs. Should it occur when your dog is standing up on only the hind legs, he will fall down and possibly seriously injure either his leg or some other part of his body.

Swimming is one of the greatest of all physical activities. It exercises almost every major muscle of the body, improves heart and breathing function, and is exhilarating to both dog and owner. If you have access to a swimming facility where you can take your dog—a fresh water stream or lake, your own swimming pool, even the ocean—you have one more experience you can share with your canine companion well into his advanced years. Once again, this assumes your veterinarian has put no medical constraints on this form of exercise and pleasure.

NUTRITION

When dogs were wild, or at least still hunted for their food, hunger may have been an occasional concern, but rarely were nutritional deficiencies or imbalances ever a problem. Dogs killed and ate almost all of their prey's carcass including the entrails, skin, and even bones. Domesticated and dependent upon their owners for food, today's dogs are amply fed, right to the point of obesity, yet they often develop a number of deficiencies from their improperly balanced diets. The advent over the past decade of nutritionally "complete" or "balanced" commercial dog foods, and their increasing acceptance by dog owners and veterinarians alike, has drastically reduced the incidence of dietary deficiencies. Today such nutritional problems are seen mostly in dogs who are fed homemade diets or a diet of table scraps and leftovers.

Poor nutrition, whether from dietary deficiencies or excesses, has a significantly negative effect on your dog's ability to remain in good health. Resistance to infection is lowered, as is the production of antibodies, allowing infectious agents to multiply rapidly and spread. The resulting fever, diarrhea, or other manifestations of illness, more than likely will make your dog less interested in eating, thus increasing the state of malnutrition. Improper nutrition also interferes with and slows the body's healing processes following surgery. It is therefore important that you provide your geriatric dog with the best available diet so as to keep her in a state of ideal nutrition. If she has lived this many years on a stable diet and is in good health, you have most likely been providing such ideal nutrition. During periods of recovery from sickness or surgery, or during other times of stress, your veterinarian may recommend increasing certain nutrients in that diet to make up for the increased demands of tissue repair.

Two statements frequently heard among human nutritionists, physicians, and social service groups are "More is known about the nutritional needs of dogs than of people," and "Most dogs in the United States are better fed than many American children." To a large degree the former is certainly true, and I suppose the latter statement has some validity in underdeveloped or underprivileged rural and urban areas. There has been, over the past thirty-plus years, a tremendous amount of research into the nutritional requirements of puppy and adult as well as reproducing and lactating dogs. Substantial research has also been conducted into the dietary needs of adult or older dogs with kidney, liver, heart, or intestinal disease. However, there has been a dearth of specific research into the needs of aging and geriatric dogs who are *in good health*. This may be due, in part, to the fact that, until this decade, precious few dogs reached old age without one or more of the aforementioned disorders. Today we see increasing numbers of dogs past twelve or fourteen whose kidneys, liver, heart, and digestive systems are relatively normal. It is hoped that this will stimulate canine nutritionists to do some research on such dogs, so we may have factual information on what healthy older dogs need in terms of nutrition. Until then, we must work with the very limited factual data available and the intuitive and experiential data provided by veterinarians involved in the care of aged dogs.

There are a few generalizations we can work with, but I must emphasize that they are *generalizations* that can vary from dog to dog. Your family veterinarian will be able to determine to what extent they are applicable to your dog. Partly because of normal aging changes in metabolism, and partly due to the usual decrease in physical activity, older dogs need fewer calories to provide adequate energy than do younger ones. This should be accomplished by reducing the *total* amount of food intake. Failure to do so will sooner or later result in an obese dog, as the unused and unneeded calories are converted into, and stored as, fat. The same normal aging changes also diminish both the absorption of certain nutrients from the intestine and the utilization of others when they are absorbed. Also protein building within body cells is substantially less efficient in aged dogs, particularly in the liver and the muscles.

The special dietary needs of dogs with particular ailments are discussed with those ailments in Part Two of this book.

For the aging dog with normal, functioning kidneys, liver, and other organs, there is little need to change from whatever diet has kept him in that state of good health, except to reduce the total amount of food per day. Some older dogs begin to have difficulty digesting large amounts of fat, so it may be desirable to reduce the daily fat intake to the minimum that will supply adequate calories and the essential fatty acids. It is often difficult to determine in an otherwise healthy dog just when these changes in absorption and utilization start. For this reason many doctors recommend the use of a vitamin-mineral supplement but these should always be complete and balanced preparations. The use of single vitamins or minerals, without their "colleagues" to balance them in the various metabolic processes, can itself produce disease. The only exception to this is if there exists a specific deficiency of a particular vitamin or mineral. These elements rarely work by themselves, but rather as a carefully balanced team, such as vitamins A, D, and E, the numerous B-vitamins, calcium and phosphorus, and other such groupings. Giving more of one than of the others, in the absence of a deficit in that one element, upsets nature's balance, and the body reacts with attempts to restore that balance or by disease.

Diet Essentials

In order to maintain life, dogs need a source of energy, amino acids, fatty acids, vitamins, minerals, and water. Although dogs consume large quantities of carbohydrates daily, no minimum requirement or even its essentiality has yet been established. It is possible to feed a dog a carbohydrate-free diet and still maintain good health as long as adequate quantities of all other nutrients are present. Normally, however, most of the daily energy needs come from dietary carbohydrate, some from fat, and less from protein. Since approximately nine calories are supplied by each gram of fat consumed, as opposed to four calories for each gram of carbohydrate or protein, it follows that less fat is needed to provide caloric energy.

Amino Acids

Amino acids are the building blocks from which proteins are made. Of the many amino acids which exist, nine are considered *essential* in the dog and must be present somewhere in the diet, as your dog cannot manufacture them within his body. These essential amino acids are:

histidine	lysine	threonine
isoleucine	methionine	tryptophan
leucine	phenylalanine	valine

A tenth, arginine, is probably also essential, but this has not yet been conclusively proven. Not all proteins contain all these amino acids, and those which do can vary in the proportions of each. Proteins which do supply all in the ideal proportions are said to have a high *biological value* and are used most efficiently by your dog's body. They are also more readily digestible, reducing the amount of protein end products his kidneys must process. Other proteins have lower biological value, more end products, and are less desirable. Muscle meats, fish, chicken, and eggs are among the ideal proteins while "meat-by-products" and plant proteins are of lower biological value.

(A word about eggs before I go further. Egg *yolks* are one of the best of all sources of protein, being of very high biological value. However, egg *whites* contain a specific protein called *avidin*, which attaches to *biotin*, an essential B-vitamin, in the digestive tract and prevents the vitamin's absorption. The possible resultant biotin deficiency is sometimes referred to as "egg-white injury." Cooking the egg may diminish this problem somewhat, but for the aging dog I advise the egg be separated and the white not be fed at all. Soft boiling also reduces the chance of mechanical digestive upset seen in some dogs when fed raw egg yolks.)

Fat

Fat in the diet, made up of many types of saturated and unsaturated fatty acids, provides the most readily available source of calories for energy but must also supply certain specific fatty acids—the *essential* ones. These are the polyunsaturates called linoleic acid, linolenic acid, and arachidonic acid, with linoleic being the most vital as your dog's body can effectively convert it into the other two. They are important in maintaining the health and integrity of the skin and other epithelial tissue, as well as in the transport of the fat-soluble vitamins—A, D, E, and K.

Carbohydrates

Carbohydrates form the bulk of most dog diets and are readily digested by the healthy canine, supplying mainly energy calories and the source from which vital blood glucose (sugar) can be manufactured. Cereals, breads, corn, and potatoes are good sources which also supply small amounts of protein. Carbohydrates are important in the normal diet as they provide readily available calories for energy, as do fats, so that proteins can be used solely for the building and rebuilding of body tissue. A dog who is deficient in carbohydrates will "burn" his proteins to provide calories. This will not only interfere with healing and tissue repair but will also place an additional burden on the kidneys to excrete the increased end products of such protein metabolism. This is something you surely don't want in your older dog even if his kidneys are still functioning more or less normally.

Minerals

The mineral requirements, in terms of amounts, are still a gray area in canine nutrition. Much of the information available has been guess-stimated or else extrapolated from research done on animals other than dogs. However, there is good evidence as to *which* minerals are needed while others are still controversial and require further study.

Required Minerals

Calcium	Iodine	Manganese	Selenium
Chlorine	Iron	Phosphorus	Sodium
Copper	Magnesium	Potassium	Zinc

Probably Required Minerals

Chromium	Fluorine	Nickel	Tin
Cobalt	Molybdenum	Silicon	Vanadium

Minerals are needed in very small to almost infinitesimal amounts per day, and exceeding these needs for any prolonged period can result in severe abnormalities of bone, heart, and kidneys among others. Mineral supplementation should be given your aging dog only on the advice of your veterinarian. It may be recommended in certain types of musculoskeletal disorders, cardiac arrhythmias, or kidney failure. Because the aging dog's bones are frequently undergoing demineralization the commonest recommended supplement is calcium and phosphorous in a proportion of 1.2 to 1.

Vitamins

Most vitamins enhance the rate of specific metabolic processes and, once again, certain ones are essential to normal life. These are the fat soluble vitamins—A, D, E, and K; and the water soluble B-vitamins—thiamine, riboflavin, pantothenic acid, niacin, piridoxine, folic acid, biotin, choline, and B-12. Vitamin C is also vitally important for good health but, because a normal healthy dog is quite capable of manufacturing ample quantities of that vitamin within its own body, there is no need for the diet to supply it. Your geriatric dog who has been fed a well-balanced diet all these years is unlikely to develop any vitamin deficiencies, even allowing for her somewhat altered ability to absorb and use them. However, when disease requires the use of special diets, which for medical reasons cannot be as complete as before, your family veterinarian may recommend the use of vitamin supplements. Follow her advice explicitly, as many vitamins are quite toxic when given in amounts significantly greater than your dog's body needs or can utilize.

Water

Perhaps the most important of all essential nutrients is *water*. Its presence is indispensable for the normal function of all living cells, yet many people do not take it into consideration when planning proper nutrition for their dogs. Unlike camels, dogs cannot store water, and any significant reduction in its intake can result in varying degrees of poor health, sickness, and even death. An "average" adult dog's body is made up of sixty to sixty-five percent water but that water is intimately bound within the cells and tissues of that body and must remain relatively constant in amount. As long as water is readily available, the normal dog will drink enough to replace whatever amount is lost through the myriad of metabolic reactions continually going on, as well as that lost through urine production. In those unusual situations where free access at all times cannot be provided, fresh water must be given a minimum of three or four times a day, spread out over the entire waking day.

The amount of each of the nutrients your dog needs, as established by the Committee on Animal Nutrition of the National Research Council, can be found by referring to the Appendix. There is no way, however, that a book can tell you your geriatric dog's specific caloric requirement. This, of needs, must vary from one dog to another, just as it does from one person to another, and is affected by your dog's individual state of health. A rough, ballpark figure for the "average, healthy, and active" dog beyond ten years of age would be between thirty-five and fifty calories per pound of body weight per day.

If your dog is happy with once-a-day feeding, that is fine, although most older dogs will benefit from and probably be happier with twice-a-day feeding. This can also be helpful in stimulating a waning appetite—but no treats, please—as it is important that both the diet and the feeding schedule be kept constant. Once in awhile your dog may skip a meal, or not finish it all, without necessarily being sick. Simply remove the uneaten food in twenty or thirty minutes. If he appears to be OK and subsequently eats normally at the next feeding, you have no problem unless this becomes a frequent occurrence, is accompanied by any sign of illness, or he continues to eat less and less. In any such case a visit to your veterinarian is in order.

OBESITY

There are several ailments which humans share with their "best friend," and obesity is unfortunately one of them. Of all the nutritionally related diseases occurring in companion animal practice, it is probably the most frequently seen and can be found in dogs of all ages. However, the likelihood of occurrence increases with advancing age and decreased activity. Obesity results from eating more than the body needs for its metabolic and other activities. Put another way, more calories are being ingested than are being burned up. Or even more simply, there is greater input than outgo! While genetic and physiological factors can affect obesity, the average pet is brought to this inglorious state by his environment, which usually contains *too much food, too little exercise*, and *an indulgent owner*.

What is obesity, as if you didn't know, and even more to the point, when is a dog considered to be obese? By definition, it is the *excessive* deposition of fat in the body's adipose tissue, whose job it is to store fat. A general rule of thumb states that a dog who is fifteen percent or more above the ideal weight for his breed qualifies as an obese individual. Granted there are variations as to what is "ideal" and certainly each dog must be assessed individually. It is not so much a matter of how many pounds or kilograms, but rather *what* that weight is made up of—fat—and *where* it is distributed in the body.

Obesity is by far the most common form of malnutrition in the dog. Yes, I said *malnutrition*! That word is not limited in meaning to undernourishment and a scrawny, unthrifty looking dog. Overnourishment, which can lead to obesity as well as certain skeletal disorders, is also malnutrition. The excess energy intake is stored as fat and can come only from food. Obesity is a serious health hazard! Caloric requirements tend to vary inversely with both age and body size, so it logically follows that the problem is more common in older dogs. Illogically, however, there seems to be no limitation to the size of the canine that becomes overweight. I have observed this hazard to good health in both Chihuahuas and Irish wolfhounds and in all sizes of dogs in between.

It is rare indeed that obesity results from an endocrine malfunction, yet many an owner of an overweight dog is convinced that there is something wrong with the dog's "glands," that it has a hormonal problem. Because our dogs live in such close proximity to us, their way of life tends to mimic our behavior closely. Two results of our modern society are a drastic curtailment of regular exercise and the availability of an abundance of food—high calorie food—especially in large metropolitan areas. It is only a short step further to obesity. Show me an obese owner, and almost always there will be an obese dog at the other end of the leash!

To most of us, obesity is not an attractive word. Overweight people do not like to hear it applied to themselves, and owners of overweight dogs don't like it applied to their pet any better. We have all heard maxims such as these or their equivalents—"you can dig your grave very quickly with your teeth"—"the bigger the belly the shorter the life"—"the most important muscles to exercise are the ones with which you push away from the dinner table." Obesity can cause, add to, or compound many other health problems and make it more difficult to deal with cardiovascular, musculoskeletal, and metabolic disorders. Obese dogs often have difficulties in locomotion, finding it uncomfortable to walk any, but short distances. All that fat in the abdomen presses forward against the diaphragm making it more arduous a task for the dog to inhale, fully expand its lungs and provide a proper exchange of air in them. As a result, these dogs seem to run out of breath with only minimal activity.

An obese animal puts a very heavy burden on the joints of its limbs, which may cause, or at least predispose it to, joint injury and disease. This is usually painful and will incline the dog to move about less. If food intake is not reduced, greater obesity results. The same self-perpetuating cycle is produced as fatty infiltration of the heart muscle reduces cardiac efficiency, lowering blood oxygen levels, and making the dog tire more easily. Again, there is less activity to use up all that extra energy being ingested. Obesity can also predispose a dog to diabetes, adversely affect existing kidney disorders, and lower natural resistance to infection.

During hot weather, it is the obese dog who suffers first and most from heat stroke or heat prostration, now collectively called heat stress. I must point out in all fairness, however, at least one redeeming asset of excess fat—it does act as a very effective insulator to keep out the winter cold. But that same insulation keeps the summer heat in once it does get into the body.

Every veterinarian takes a deep breath when he sees an obese patient come into the examining room. Abdominal palpation and listening to the heart and lungs with the stethoscope are a vital part of every physical examination. Yet, because of the excess fat deposits, it is very difficult to accurately feel the individual abdominal organs and often quite impossible to hear abnormal, or even normal, heart and lung sounds. The risks inherent in the administration of anesthesia are significantly, and often dangerously, increased in the obese patient. The physical difficulty of performing surgery through such heavy pads of fat prolong the anesthetic and surgery time, making the prognosis less optimistic.

Double M is a case in point. A miniature schnauzer of smallish build, who weighed eighteen pounds at six months of age, she lives with a wonderfully cheerful and loving childless couple who themselves are quite heavy. Needless to say, every whim of this dog was indulged from the first day, including food. She was encouraged to always eat "heartily" and by the time she was three years weighed in at twenty-five pounds. Most of that weight was in her substantial abdomen. She began to show symptoms of what in most other dogs would have been a minor, short-lasting inflammation of the urinary bladder. But not Double M! Because of reduced natural resistance to infection, it developed into a difficult-to-treat bladder infection which took seven months to clear up.

Frequent discussions with the owners during the previous two years had produced no results toward reducing this schnauzer's weight. I simply couldn't convince them to stick with a proper feeding program. In fairness to these people, I must admit that Double M most assuredly knew how to turn on those sad doelike eyes when she wanted food. She used them on me many times in the examining room for other reasons.

During the time of the bladder infection she was indulged with even more food and proceeded to put on another two pounds, for a total of twenty-seven. She was soon after presented for examination because of a recently noticed difficulty in getting up from a lying position. The discomfort seemed most pronounced in her hind legs. Radiographs (X-rays) of both legs, as well as the stifle and hip joints, revealed no visible abnormalities. I read the owners the riot act and told them that Double M had to be reduced by thirty percent of her weight! Her legs simply couldn't support her great corpulence any more. Two months later she had lost *one pound* which she managed to put back on during the third month. Almost in desperation, a prescription reducing diet was advised as the sole source of food. This seemingly drastic step hit home with the owners, for they stuck to the program, and in three months Double M was down to twenty-four pounds. Then suddenly, she lost no more as snacks, tidbits, and other goodies were returned to the menu.

About a year later this friendly schnauzer developed a uterine infection—pyometra—severe enough to require an immediate ovariohysterectomy. Trying to remove even such a distended organ through all the fat that covered it, was no simple task. Everything was greasy to the touch and slipped through my fingers, as well as out of the surgical instruments, over and over again. Both surgical and anesthetic times were prolonged by at least forty percent, thereby increasing the potential dangers, and it took twice as long to suture the abdomen closed. Healing was also delayed but fortunately Double M made a satisfactory recovery. So satisfactory, in fact, that within one year she had gone back up to twenty-eight pounds. Please note carefully that this weight increase was *not* due to being "spayed," another of the myriad of old-wives' tales about the causes of obesity. Rather, it seems each of the owners felt their beloved dog needed "building up" after her operation, and each one tried to do the entire job.

Well, they sure built her up and continued to do so, despite my repeated urgings to the contrary, until at the age of eight and a half years Double M tipped the scales at *thirty* pounds! A short time later this roly-poly dog developed a cystic calculus—a stone in the urinary bladder—again requiring abdominal surgery. The riot act was read once more, and she was put on a below-maintenance diet, resulting in a loss of six pounds within two months. Nevertheless, the greasy abdominal contents still made the bladder and other organs quite slippery and troublesome to work with. Respiration was quite labored throughout the operation and necessitated frequent mechanical assistance to help fully expand the lungs against the pressure of all that fat. Perhaps Double M has the fabled "nine lives" of a cat, because she came through this threat to her health with flying colors. Three months later, as of this writing, she is healed satisfactorily, and the secondary urinary infection has cleared up. But alas, the waistline is growing again!

The most important thing you can do for obesity in your dog is to *prevent* it. Once excess fat has been deposited in the body, it is exceedingly difficult to get rid of, as the owner of any obese dog will readily tell you. It takes an awful lot of exercise to burn off just a few ounces. Nevertheless, adequate exercise, commensurate with any physical or medical limitations your aging dog may have, is an essential constituent of the prevention program. The small active dog can likely supply all necessary activity by itself, even if limited to running about in an apartment. Most other dogs will need additional directed walking and/or running. Even the outdoor or suburban dog may need some directed exercise.

As vital as all this physical activity is, however, the key to excess fat control is diet control! Total food intake for each day should provide only the number of calories your dog needs for daily living. Of course, these calories must provide properly balanced and adequate amounts of protein, carbohydrate, and fat as discussed previously in this section. Your family veterinarian will be able to tell you if your dog is in good shape. You can keep her in a desirable state by using the chart on pages 32–33, referring to the first section. Find her wieght in pounds or kilograms, and determine the number of calories she requires each day (your veterinarian may advise a lower caloric requirement, based on your dog's individual differences). Adjacent to that number you will find the weight needed, in grams, of the type food you are feeding to provide the required calories. All dog food packages should now give weights in metric measure so there will be no need for elaborate calculations. (In the event they are not so given on your brand of food, you will find a conversion table in Appendix IV.) For those of you who are still feeding homemade diets, the U.S. Department of Agriculture publishes "Composition of Foods," Agricultural Handbook number 8, at a cost of less than four dollars, which gives the caloric value of most common and not-so-common foods.

It is a good idea to weigh your dog at home, always on the same scale and at about the same time of the day, at least once every three months to be sure her weight is staying where you want it to be. This can very easily be done by weighing yourself first, then picking up your dog and weighing the both of you. The difference in the two readings is your dog's weight. If you happen to own one of the larger breeds and cannot possibly lift Duchess up, you will have to find a commercial scale with a platform large enough for her to stand on. Fluctuations, up or down, of five percent of her total weight should be of no concern, unless they happen with unexpected suddenness, or they continue in one direction only.

The data in the chart on pages 32–33 refer to the "normal" or "average" dog, and are based upon statistics obtained from many hundreds of test dogs. But we all know that your dog, or anyone else's for that matter, is not "average." Wide variations can be found between different breeds and between individuals within a breed. An old, but still active, Lakeland terrier may indeed use up as many calories as the "average" dog. On the other hand, the mature cocker spaniel who curls up in the armchair most of the day, or the aged German shepherd who lies on the soft carpet near the radiator or in front of the fireplace and has to be prodded to any kind of activity, surely needs far less food intake. Your veterinarian will have to guide you in the use of these "normal" statistics and you should consult with him or her *before* you make any sudden change in your dog's diet.

If much to your dismay, your dog has the misfortune already to be obese—what do you do now? Quickie diets rarely keep the excess weight off any longer in dogs than they do in people. It requires the slow, continual removal of extra fat in order to become

RECOMMENDED DAILY INTAKE FOR NORMAL AND OVERWEIGHT ADULT DOGS

Weight / Intake		I. Normal Adult Maintenance				II. Caloric Restriction 10%				III. Caloric Restriction 20%			
1	2	3	4	5	6	7	8	9	10	11	12	13	14
Body Weight Of Dog Kg	Lb	Gross Energy Calories	Dry Dog Food ( )=cups Grams	Semi-Moist Dog Food ( )=packets Grams	Canned Dog Food ( )=cans Grams	Gross Energy Calories	Dry Dog Food ( )=cups Grams	Semi-Moist Dog Food ( )=packets Grams	Canned Dog Food ( )=cans Grams	Gross Energy Calories	Dry Dog Food ( )=cups Grams	Semi-Moist Dog Food ( )=packets Grams	Canned Dog Food ( )=cans Grams
1	2.2	165.0	37.8	41.9	113.0	148.5	34.1	37.7	101.7	132.0	30.3	33.5	90.4
2	4.4	277.5	63.6	70.4	190.1	249.7	57.3	63.4	171.1	222.0	50.9	56.3	152.1
3	6.6	376.1	86.3	95.5	257.6	338.5	77.6	85.9	231.9	300.9	69.0	76.4	206.1
4	8.8	466.7	107.0(1)	118.4	319.7	420.0	96.3	106.6	287.7	373.4	85.6	94.8	255.7
5	11.0	551.7	126.5	140.0	377.9	496.5	113.9(1)	126.0	340.1	441.4	101.2(1)	112.0	302.3
6	13.2	632.6	145.1	160.5(1)	433.3(1)	569.3	130.6	144.5	389.9	506.0	116.1	128.4	346.6
7	15.4	710.1	162.9	180.2	486.4	639.1	146.6	162.2	437.7(1)	568.1	130.3	144.2	389.1
8	17.6	784.9	180.0	199.2	537.6	706.4	162.0	179.3(1)	483.8	627.9	144.0	159.4	430.1
9	19.8	857.4	196.6	217.6	587.2	771.6	177.0	195.8	528.5	685.9	157.3	174.1(1)	469.8(1)
10	22.0	927.9	212.8(2)	235.5	635.5	835.1	191.5	211.9	572.0	742.3	170.3	188.4	508.4
11	24.3	996.6	228.6	252.9	682.6	897.0	205.7(2)	227.7	614.4	797.3	182.9	202.4	546.1
12	26.5	1063.8	244.0	270.0	728.6	957.4	219.6	243.0	655.8	851.1	195.2	216.0	582.9
13	28.7	1129.6	259.1	286.7	773.7	1016.7	233.2	258.0	696.4	903.7	207.3(2)	229.4	619.0
14	30.9	1194.2	273.9	303.1	818.0	1074.8	246.5	272.8	736.2	955.4	219.1	242.5	654.4
15	33.1	1257.6	288.4	319.2	861.4(2)	1131.9	259.6	287.3	775.3	1006.1	230.8	255.4	689.1
16	35.3	1320.0	302.8(3)	335.0	904.1	1188.0	272.5	301.5	813.7	1056.0	242.2	268.0	723.3
17	37.5	1381.4	316.8	350.6(2)	946.2	1243.3	285.2	315.5	851.6	1105.1	253.5	280.5	756.9
18	39.7	1441.9	330.7	366.0	987.6	1297.7	297.6	329.4	888.8(2)	1153.5	264.6	292.8	790.1
19	41.9	1501.6	344.4	381.1	1028.5	1351.4	310.0(3)	343.0(2)	925.6	1201.3	275.5	304.9	822.8

20	**44.1**	1560.5	357.9	396.1	1068.8	1404.4	322.1	356.5	961.9	1248.4	286.3	316.8	855.1(2)
21	**46.3**	1618.6	371.2	410.8	1108.7	1456.8	334.1	369.7	997.8	1294.9	297.0(3)	328.7	886.9
22	**48.5**	1676.1	384.4	425.4	1148.0	1508.5	346.0	382.9	1033.2	1340.9	307.5	340.3(2)	918.4
23	**50.7**	1732.9	397.5(4)	439.8	1186.9	1559.6	357.7	395.8	1068.2	1386.3	318.0	351.9	949.5
24	**52.9**	1789.1	410.4	454.1	1225.4	1610.2	369.3	408.7	1102.9	1431.3	328.3	363.3	980.3
25	**55.1**	1844.8	423.1	468.2	1263.5	1660.3	380.8	421.4	1137.2	1475.2	338.5	374.6	1010.8
26	**57.3**	1899.8	435.7	482.2	1301.3(3)	1709.8	392.2(4)	434.0	1171.1	1519.9	348.6	385.8	1041.0
27	**59.5**	1954.4	448.2	496.0(3)	1338.6	1758.9	403.4	446.4	1204.7	1563.5	358.6	396.8	1070.9
28	**61.7**	2008.4	460.6	509.7	1375.6	1807.6	414.6	458.8	1238.1	1606.7	368.5	407.8	1100.5
29	**63.9**	2062.0	472.9	523.3	1412.3	1855.8	425.6	471.0	1271.1	1649.6	378.3	418.7	1129.8
30	**66.1**	2115.1	485.1	536.8	1448.7	1903.6	436.6	483.1	1303.8(3)	1692.1	388.1	429.5	1158.9
31	**68.3**	2167.7	497.2(5)	550.2	1484.7	1951.0	447.5	495.2	1336.3	1734.2	397.7(4)	440.1	1187.8
32	**70.5**	2220.0	509.2	563.4	1520.5	1998.0	458.2	507.1(3)	1368.5	1776.0	407.3	450.8	1216.4
33	**72.8**	2271.8	521.1	576.6	1556.0	2044.6	468.9	518.9	1400.4	1817.4	416.8	461.3	1244.8
34	**75.0**	2323.2	532.9	589.7	1591.3	2090.9	479.6	530.7	1432.1	1858.6	426.3	471.7	1273.0
35	**77.2**	2374.3	544.6	602.6	1626.2	2136.9	490.1	542.4	1463.6	1899.4	435.7	482.1	1301.0(3)
36	**79.4**	2425.0	556.2	615.5	1661.0	2182.5	500.6(5)	553.9	1494.9	1940.0	445.0	492.4	1328.8
37	**81.6**	2475.3	567.7	628.3	1695.4	2227.8	511.0	565.4	1525.9	1980.3	454.2	502.6	1356.4
38	**83.8**	2525.4	579.2	641.0	1729.7(4)	2272.8	521.3	576.9	1556.7	2020.3	463.4	512.8(3)	1383.8
39	**86.0**	2575.0	590.6	653.6	1763.7	2317.5	531.5	588.2	1587.3	2060.0	472.5	522.8	1411.0
40	**88.2**	2624.4	601.9(6)	666.1	1797.5	2362.0	541.7	599.5	1617.8	2099.5	481.5	532.9	1438.0
41	**90.4**	2673.4	613.2	678.5(4)	1831.1	2406.1	551.9	610.7	1648.0	2138.8	490.5	542.8	1464.9
42	**92.6**	2722.2	624.4	690.9	1864.5	2450.0	561.9	621.8	1678.1	2177.8	499.5(5)	552.7	1491.6
43	**94.8**	2770.7	635.5	703.2	1897.7	2493.6	571.9	632.9	1707.9	2216.5	508.4	562.6	1518.2
44	**97.0**	2818.9	646.5	715.4	1930.7	2537.0	581.9	643.9	1737.7(4)	2255.1	517.2	572.4	1544.6
45	**99.2**	2866.8	657.5	727.6	1963.5	2580.1	591.8	654.8	1767.2	2293.4	526.0	582.1	1570.8
46	**101.4**	2914.4	668.4	739.7	1996.2	2623.0	601.6(6)	665.7	1796.6	2331.5	534.8	591.8	1596.9
47	**103.6**	2961.8	679.3	751.7	2028.6	2665.6	611.4	676.6(4)	1825.8	2369.4	543.5	601.4	1622.9
48	**105.8**	3008.9	690.1	763.7	2060.9	2708.1	621.1	687.3	1854.8	2407.2	552.1	611.0	1648.7
49	**108.0**	3055.8	700.9(7)	775.6	2093.0	2750.3	630.8	698.0	1883.7	2444.7	560.7	620.5	1674.4
50	**110.2**	3102.5	711.6	787.4	2125.0(5)	2792.2	640.4	708.7	1912.5	2482.0	569.3	629.9	1700.0(4)

Courtesy of The Quaker Oats Company.

stable over the long haul. The reducing of an obese dog, as with an obese person, should not be undertaken without a thorough medical examination first. There may be other health factors which could be adversely affected by too rapid a weight loss. You and your family veterinarian must work together as a team in order to effect a successful and safe weight reduction in your dog. It is vital that you believe in and be totally committed to the desirability of succeeding in this project and be motivated sufficiently to withstand the temptations, both from yourself and your dog, to stray from the established diet. *All* snacks, tidbits, rewards and other such goodies must be eliminated during the reducing period. For the canine who has been allowed to become a glutton, it may be necessary to divide the day's total ration into several small feedings spread out over the day. Even the nonglutton should have its total ration divided into two feedings. Of course, the outdoor dog must be prevented from raiding the garbage can or otherwise scavenging.

Depending upon how motivated, cooperative, and dependable you are, your veterinarian may advise changing only the amount of your dog's present basic diet. If you have been feeding table scraps and leftovers, you will have to change to a more predictable and constant diet, and he may recommend one of the "complete nutrition" commercial dog foods. He will discuss with you the dog's estimated degree of obesity, and together you will decide what a proper and *realistic* weight for her should be. The total daily caloric intake will be determined as if she already were that weight, and by feeding only that amount she will slowly lose fat. Using statistics similar to those in the table on pages 32–33, he will recommend either the number of calories or the weight of food you should feed. In the event other health problems require a slower, less radical weight reduction, refer to section III, or even II of the table. Caloric Restriction 20% and Caloric Restriction 10% will provide you with the correct calories and food amounts. You must be steadfast in not increasing the diet above the amount decided upon, no matter how sadly your dog looks at you or paws at you for extras. Certainly you must be patient—safe reducing does take time.

It will not be easy in the beginning. It can be a most difficult time for your dog, who will feel hungry because her stomach is not being filled and stretched to the same extent that used to produce a satiated feeling. It will surely be a difficult time for you. By the end of the first week you may start to see those begging eyes—and she will beg at every opportunity—everywhere you go, even in your dreams. She may follow you from room to room trying to convince you that she is surely going to starve to death. But she won't convince you—if you *really* love her—and she most certainly will not starve to death or even become remotely ill! She will in fact be able to live significantly longer than she would have, had she continued to be obese. That will give you more time in which to share your life and love with her. Anything worth doing is worth doing well, we have all been taught. Attaining a safe and healthy weight is something very worth doing and leaves no room for compromise.

There will probably be little noticeable change in weight for one to two weeks, but then you will be able to appreciate that the fat is slowly, but surely, coming off. Keep a written record of her weight all through the reducing period, weighing her every third day for the first two weeks (so you won't get discouraged) and daily from then on. Success may be achieved in only a few weeks, or it may take many months, depending on the amount of loss being undertaken.

Should you find it emotionally or otherwise difficult to stick to your guns, or if you're a pushover for those pleading eyes, there are special reducing diets available on prescription that allow for some overindulgence by you. The trouble is that they are not very palatable, and many dogs simply won't eat them. Now that would be fine for a while—there's no faster way to reduce than to not eat at all—but that is not the healthiest way to do it. Besides, you surely wouldn't let your dog skip more than a meal or two, at most, before you'd go right back to her regular food at her regular amount (that's to make up for all those meals she skipped) and we're right back where we started! It is sometimes possible to add bulky low calorie fillers to a reducing diet, so your dog will feel more satisfied, but these must be used with great care and only on the advice of your veterinarian.

Commitment and perseverance will bring the reward of a dog who once again has that trim and fit look of good health, minus the many hazards of being obese! Eventually the day will come when your dog does reach the desired weight. She will no longer be chasing you around the house looking for food, because her stomach now will not need such large amounts of food to make her feel "full." She may, on the other hand, be chasing you because, for the first time in many years, she feels good enough to bounce around and be playful. If your fit and trim dog continues to lose weight below the desired level, you will increase the amount of food—the *same* kind of food, unless it was a prescription diet—by a *small* amount, bit by bit, a little at a time until the desired weight is reached and then kept there.

It is hoped that the recollection of what it took, on the part of both you and your dog, to eliminate obesity will successfully prevent you from ever allowing that unhealthy, inglorious state to recur!

GROOMING

Proper and effective grooming contributes only indirectly to your dog's general health but becomes a more significant factor with increasing age. As the natural skin oils come to be less effecttively produced, the skin can become dry and scaly, causing itchiness and discomfort. Matted or tangled haircoats likewise cause scratching and, in addition, can hold dirt and debris on the skin from which bacteria can readily enter skin that is already abraded by the scratching and chewing. Bacterial dermatitis is not at all uncommon in older dogs.

The daily grooming patterns begun in earlier years should be continued throughout a dog's lifetime. It is my firm belief that all dogs, with the possible exception of some show dogs and those with certain skin diseases, should be combed and brushed *every day* of their lives with a metal comb and a *wire*-bristle slicker-type brush (Twinco makes a very good one). Combing should be done first, as its purpose is merely to remove tangles and separate the hairs so the slicker brush does not get caught in them. This is followed by the brush which should be used in firmly applied, long, slow strokes. The object of the brushing is to get the wires down to the skin, which is where the dirt is, to remove that dirt and the dry scales of dead skin. A well-made brush, such as the Twinco, will not scratch or irritate the skin as long as it is kept parallel to the skin at all times, following the natural curves of the body, and moved in the same direction as the lay of the hair. Because the individual wires of the brush are bent at mid-shaft and set into a rubber pad, they flex readily and act like your fingers do when you are massaging your scalp. Your dog will be aware of, and feel, the brush, but it will not hurt him.

There are exceptions, of course, to this routine. Chihuahuas and other very short-haired dogs should be brushed daily but with less pressure applied to the brush. Obviously a comb is not needed with these canines. If your dog has skin tumors or warts, you must carefully avoid them with both comb and brush. It is quite easy to tear off small warts and cause bleeding. Should this occur, place a small peice of absorbent cotton on the wound and press firmly on it with your finger for five minutes by the clock. This will stop the bleeding from almost all such wounds. It is also possible to use a carefully applied styptic pencil, but be certain to hold your dog firmly—it often stings!

My beliefs concerning bathing of a dog are also somewhat less than conventional. Assuming you do brush *effectively* every day, it is not necessary to bathe a dog at all, unless it falls into a mudhole or there are medical reasons for doing so. Even city dogs can be kept clean by daily grooming alone and will have very little, if any, odor. Frequent bathing over-softens the haircoat, removes natural skin oils, and produces drying of the skin and a dull coat. If you have a white dog, you may have to settle for an off-white in the pollution of the big city, where nothing short of weekly or more frequent bathing will keep a white dog really white. Nevertheless, if you feel you must bathe your aging dog—and I recognize that many dog owners have this need—there are some precautions to be taken.

First, make certain the surface your dog will stand on during the bath is not slippery. Good footing, such as a rubber mat indoors or pavement or grass outdoors, will prevent mishaps that could easily result in injuries to the more brittle bones and less resilient joints and muscles of your senior citizen. Before wetting her, place cotton into each ear canal to keep the shampoo and bath water out of her ears. Failure to do so can precipitate ear problems, as the lining of the canal, like the body's skin, has with age become less resistant to minor irritants. For similar reasons a drop of clean mineral or olive oil or a bland non-cortisone eye ointment should be placed in each eye. Of course, remember to remove the protective ear cotton when the bath is over and your dog is dried.

Drying should be done quite thoroughly, even in summertime, with towels or a cautiously used portable hair dryer. Be sure to dry the feet, especially under and between the toe pads. Damp hair will readily pick up debris from the ground and hold it. This may prompt the dog to lick excessively at the feet, trying to dry them and remove the debris, and it can lead to interdigital (between the toes) dermatitis. In cool weather, bathing should be done indoors, and the dog not allowed out again until the following morning, so do it at night. Finally, if you must bathe your dog, please do it as infrequently as possible, and ask your veterinarian to recommend a shampoo which he knows is less likely to remove skin oils.

I have had many clients bring dogs to me for the first time and, after explaining my recommendations about daily grooming and no bathing, say that no one ever suggested anything like it, or else that they completely disagree with me. With few exceptions, however, everyone who followed my recommendations for at least four to eight weeks reported that their dog's coat became clean, glossy, almost like new and, most important, healthier even when minor skin disorders had previously been present.

One of the most common grooming problems seen in older dogs is overgrown toenails. This is particularly true of apartment, or other mostly indoor dogs. For some reason many owners think the nails need less frequent trimming as their dog grows older. Toenails grow at a fairly constant rate throughout life and for a time after death. When your dog stands squarely on all fours in a normal stance, the toenails should just touch the ground. If they are longer they will tend to bend the toes upward, often to such a degree as to cause discomfort, pain, or lameness.

Special attention must be given to the dewclaws if they are still present. These are remnants of what used to be a thumb and, because they never reach the ground surface, do not wear down at all. They can grow completely around in a circle, penetrate into the toe or foot and cause pain, infection, or abscess. The same is true, to a lesser degree, of all overgrown toenails. Nail trimming

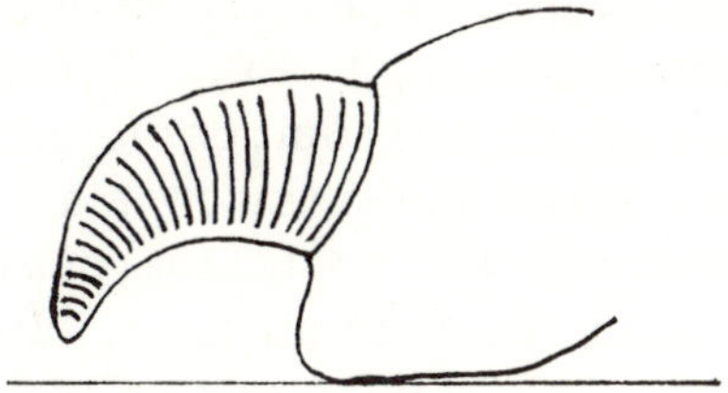

Normal toenail

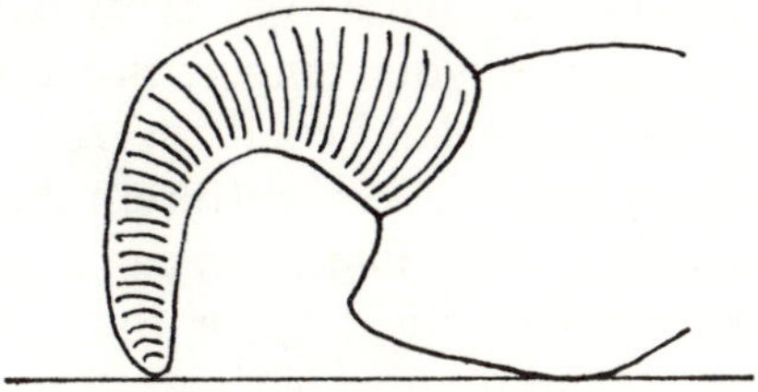

Overgrown toenail

should be done by you and done regularly. I prefer the Resco-type nail trimmer, while others may like the open style found in the White's nail trimmer. Whichever is easier for you to use should be your choice.

If you have not yet learned how to trim your dog's toenails, ask your groomer or your veterinarian to show you. Inasmuch as most veterinarians no longer do grooming, they may not trim the nails for you but, during a regular office visit, I'm sure they will demonstrate the technique to you on one or two nails.

All male dogs have a slight but frequent discharge coming from their prepuce, the soft tube skin covering the penis, which they normally keep clean by themselves. As they mature and lose some of the backbone flexibility which allows them to reach this area, they may not clean it often enough, and the hairs at the tip of the prepuce can become matted and odorous. This is especially likely in dogs with heavy coats and very long preputial hairs. Soaking with a warm, *plain water* compress until the caked hairs separate, then combing and washing the entire area with plain water, will remove the debris most of the time. Do not use soap in this area, as the opening of the prepuce is very sensitive to irritation. The overlong preputial hairs may be trimmed back to a length of one inch beyond the tip of the prepuce, but no shorter. This area of frequent soiling should be checked daily when you brush your male dog's abdomen.

As part of your dog's daily grooming routine, you should also wipe out the inner corners of his eyes with a bit of dry cotton. This will prevent the unsightly accumulation and matting of the normal eye secretions, usually referred to as "sleepers." Ears should similarly be wiped out every day using a piece of dry cotton over the end of your finger, not a cotton-tipped applicator. Be sure your finger nail is well covered. The anatomy and contour of your dog's ears are very different than yours, and unless you are really familiar with them, you can create problems with applicator sticks by injuring the wall of the ear canal or the eardrum itself. My physician used to tell me, "Don't put anything into your ear that is smaller than your elbow!" and I agree in principle with his concept. By cleaning the ears daily, you remove the tiny amounts of normally produced wax and prevent most ear problems. Should a problem develop anyway, you will know about it right away before it has time to become a serious one.

IMMUNIZATION

Regular preventive immunization against the major infectious diseases of canines has been, and will continue to be, a vital contributing factor in helping your dog reach his senior years free from the ravages of canine distemper, infectious canine hepatitis, leptospirosis, and rabies.

It is a common belief among many otherwise well-informed dog owners that distemper and hepatitis are diseases that affect only puppies or young dogs. Nothing could be farther from the truth! The viruses which cause these diseases are not respecters of maturity—only of effective immunization. Dogs of any age are susceptible, if they have not been properly vaccinated or if their antibody titer (level of immunity) is allowed to fall below a certain protective level, specific for each disease, by the absence of timely booster vaccinations. The level of immune response reaches its peak shortly after the administration of the vaccine and remains there for many months. The duration of this peak level time, and the rate at which it declines, vary from dog to dog. In most canines antibody titer will not fall below the minimum protective level for upwards of one year for distemper and hepatitis, shorter for leptospirosis, and longer for rabies. However, a small number may lose their protection in less than one year, while others will remain well protected for two years or more, depending upon the degree of natural exposure.

Booster injections for distemper and hepatitis should be given every year and would normally be administered at the time of the annual geriatric exam, unless regional or seasonal variations dictate another time of year. It is recommended that a modified live virus vaccine be used, as it stimulates the highest degree of antibody response your dog is capable of producing. Dead virus vaccines have recently been introduced which claim to stimulate an equally high response. The final choice of the particular vaccine to be used should be left to your family veterinarian.

Until recently booster injections for leptospirosis were given each year along with the distemper and hepatitis boosters, all three being combined in a single injection—the 3 in 1, or DHL. It has been shown, however, that protective levels against leptospirosis are probably not maintained for more than four to six months, and recently there have been reports of an occasional serious hypersensitivity reaction with its use. If leptospirosis is common in your area, booster injections should be given two or three times a year. On the other hand, if there is no significant incidence of the disease, many veterinarians are now recommending that boosters for it not be given at all.

All mammals are susceptible to the virus of rabies regardless of age. If a rabid bat or fox or cat bites your unprotected dog, and virus is passed, your dog will very likely develop a case of rabies whether he is six months, two, ten, or eighteen years old. The notion that a dog no longer needs rabies vaccination when he gets beyond "x" number of years is simply not correct. Granted an older dog may become less active and perhaps be less likely to be exposed; but unless your dog is going to live his remaining years in "glass house" confinement, there is still a very real chance of his meeting an infected animal. Even apartment-house dogs go outdoors and, with the increased ease with which canines can travel—from city to farm, from suburban to urban areas, from a rabies-endemic to a rabies-free area—the disease can readily be spread. Rabies is once more on the rise in many parts of the United States, because it has gotten into the wild animal population—skunks, foxes, wolves, raccoons, etc. In addition, there have been disturbing though rare reports of rabies being produced, like the human common cold, by airborne transmission instead of by an animal bite!

There are several types of rabies vaccines available, each producing a different duration of protection. Most modified live virus products will protect for three years, although two are effective for only one year. Of the pair of dead vaccines currently available, one offers good protection for three years, the other only for one. Unless there are special reasons to choose otherwise, such as foreign travel or possible medical reasons requiring a specific vaccine, a modified live virus rabies vaccination should be given your aging dog every three years for his entire lifetime. Again, the choice of the particular vaccine should be left to your family veterinarian.

Booster Vaccination Schedule for the Aging Dog

Canine distemper	Annually
Infectious canine hepatitis	Annually
Rabies	Every three years
Leptospirosis	Two or three times a year

(only in areas where leptospirosis is common)

Many functions of the canine body can become sluggish, less efficient, or inactive with advancing age. Changes in metabolism, immune response, ability to utilize proteins, etc., can have considerable effects on the level of immunity. This can result in the protective level falling more rapidly in our senior dogs than would be expected in a younger one. Once-yearly boosters for distemper and hepatitis should still be able to protect most older dogs adequately. However, show dogs, performing dogs, and all others which have frequent contact with large numbers of other canines and are subjected to the stresses therefrom, should be given booster vaccinations at least twice a year and, in some instances, before each such contact. As far as is known, it is not possible to overimmunize your dog, so don't take any unnecessary chances.

THE ANNUAL EXAMINATION

The concept of preventive veterinary medicine, other than regular immunization, is not new, but it has come to the fore in the past fifteen or twenty years. As the major killers of thirty and forty years ago—distemper, hepatitis, auto injuries—were brought under control, both the veterinarian and dog owner have been able to look at the dog's overall health preventively. Well into the fifties most veterinarians were treating dogs who were already sick. Today we still treat lots of sick dogs, but an increasing part of our daily patient load is made up of preventive examinations, diagnostics, and consultations. We all know the old adage "an ounce of prevention is worth a pound of cure." It is just as true today as when it was first spoken. Would that all of us applied it to our pets as well as to ourselves.

Perhaps the single, most significant, and far reaching thing you can do to insure your dog's continuing good health, insofar as that is possible, is to have your family veterinarian give him a complete, in-depth, system-by-system examination including certain basic laboratory tests. I am talking about the same kind of exam you and I should be getting every year after we reach forty. Your dog should have it done annually after the age of five.

Most dogs undergo slow subtle changes in kidney function starting at about five years of age. Though usually not apparent externally, these changes can be detected by laboratory analysis. Other organs and body systems, such as the heart, lungs, liver, bladder, eyes, and genital tract, may also show beginning signs of aging or disease. Early diagnosis can prevent or slow down deterioration of these vital life functions. Disease processes can be more effectively treated if they are detected in their early stages. This is especially true of cardiovascular disorders and malignancies which, as in people, are diagnosed more often today as life is prolonged.

In our clinic this preventive procedure is called the Annual Physical Examination and Laboratory Workup and includes, but is not limited to, the following:

- Physical Examination
    - Vital signs—temperature, pulse, and respiration
    - External organs
        - Ophthalmoscopic examination of the eyes
        - Ears and auditory canals
        - Nostrils and nasal passages
        - Oral cavity—lips, gums, teeth, tongue, pharynx, and tonsils

- External lymph nodes
- Skin and hair coat
- Anus, anal sacs, and external genitalia
- Limbs and joints
- Spinal column
- Neurological reflexes

Internal organs

- Palpation of stomach, liver, intestines, uterus, bladder, and prostate gland
- Auscultation of heart and lungs, and percussion of the lungs
- Palpation of the femoral and jugular pulses

Laboratory Workup

Urinalysis and, if indicated, bacterial culture

Blood studies

- Hematocrit
- Red cell sedimentation rate
- Total white cell count
- Differential white cell count
- Heartworm test
- Blood urea nitrogen
- Blood glucose (sugar)
- SGPT (serum glutamic pyruvate transaminase)
- SAP (serum alkaline phosphatase)

Fecal analysis

For patients in whom the above examinations so indicate, electrocardiograms, X-ray studies or other diagnostic tests may be recommended.

I've provided here the form used in our clinic for this preventive study. Your family veterinarian's procedures may vary in detail from these but will still gather essentially the same information. He may recommend chest X rays or other blood tests as a routine annual procedure. Another veterinarian may advise electrocardiograms every year. In our clinic, we suggest both heart X rays and an electrocardiogram every year after the age of ten, or in any dog with a history of cardiovascular disorder.

Regardless of the details of the examination, it will include a very careful history-taking covering diet, activity, urination and defecation patterns, immunizations, and any changes in per-

ANNUAL PHYSICAL EXAMINATION REPORT

Date____________

Owner's Name ____________ Telephone____________

Address____________ City____________ Zip Code____________

HISTORY: Pet's Name____________ Breed______ Age____ Weight____ Sex____

Illnesses____________

Water Consumption____________ Urination: Volume & Frequency____________

Stool Consistency____________ Diet____________

Temperament______ Heat Periods______ Current Medication______

Other____________

IMMUNIZATION STATUS: Date of Last Vaccination: (1) Distemper______ (2) Rabies______

(3) Hepatitis______ (4) Leptospirosis______

GENERAL: Temp.______ Pulse______ Height______ Weight______

Respiration Rate & Character____________

SKIN: Hair Coat______ Epidermis______ Parasites______ Tumors______

Hydration______ Glands and Lymph Nodes______

EYES: Eyelids______ Conjunctiva______ Nictitating Membrane______

Sclera______ Cornea______ Iris______

Anterior Chamber______ Lens______ Posterior Chamber______

Retina______ Tonometer Pressure______

NOSE: Anterior Nares______ Posterior Nares______ Discharge______

MOUTH: Gums______ Tumors______ Mucous Membranes______

Tongue______ Palate______

TEETH: Calculus______ Abscessed______ Loose______ Broken______

Retained Deciduous______ Other______

THROAT: Tonsils_____ Pharynx_____ Glands: (1) Mandibular_____

(2) Submaxilliary_____ (3) Cervical_____

Other_____

EARS: Ear Flap_____ Ear Canal_____ Tympanum (drum)_____

Parasites_____ Ulcers_____ Infection_____

Fungus_____ Foreign Bodies_____ Other_____

RESPIRATORY SYSTEM: Larynx_____ Trachea_____

Auscultation_____ Percussion_____

X-Ray, if needed_____ Other_____

CARDIO-VASCULAR SYSTEM: Rate_____ Enlargement_____ Valves_____

Abnormal Sounds_____ Electrocardiogram, if needed_____

Lymphatic System_____ Femoral Pulse_____ Circ. Time_____

ABDOMINAL CAVITY: Ascites_____ Pain_____ Tumors_____

Palpation_____ Liver_____

Spleen_____ Intestines_____

Bladder_____ Inguinal Glands_____

X-Ray, if needed_____ Other_____

LEGS: Joints_____ Soft Tissue_____ Pads_____ Nails_____

Feet_____ Deformities_____

RECTAL AREA: Anal Sacs_____ Anus_____ Prostate_____

Tail_____ Pelvis_____ Tape Segs_____

NERVOUS SYSTEM: Push Reflex_____ Pin Reflex_____ Scratch_____

Placing Reflex_____ Pain_____ Knee Jerk_____

General Equilibrium and Coordination_____

REPRODUCTIVE SYSTEM: Scrotum_____ Testes_____ Sheath & Penis_____

Vulva_____ Vagina_____

Cervix_____ Uterine Palpation_____

Mammae_____

SPINE & MUSCULO-SKELETAL: Neck_____ Dorsum_____ Tail_____

Fat Covering_____ Fleshing_____ Muscle Tone_____

Gait_____

LABORATORY TESTS

URINARY SYSTEM:

Specific Gravity______ Sugar______ Color______

Albumen______ Blood______ Casts______

Bilirubin______ pH______ Sediment______

BLOOD STUDIES:

Hematocrit: PCV______ Hbg______ WBC______ RBC______

Differential, if indicated______

Sed. Rate______ Heartworm Mico-Filaria______

Other______

BLOOD CHEMISTRY:

Glucose______ BUN______ Creatinine______

Total Protein______ Globulin______ Alb/Glob Ratio______

Alkaline Phosphatase______ Uric Acid______ SGOT______

SGPT______ BSP______ PSP______

Bilirubin: Direct______ Indirect______ Total______

Cholesterol______ Circ. Time______ Other______

INTERNAL PARASITES:

Hookworms______ Round Worms______ Whip Worms______

Tape Worms______ Coccidia______ Strongyloides______

Other______

SKIN SCRAPING:

Demodex______ Sarcoptes______ Fungi______ Woods Light______

Other______

CULTURE & SENSITIVITY:

Organism______

Sensitive to______

SUMMARY AND RECOMMENDATIONS

SUMMARY OF DISORDERS (OR EXAM): ____________________

RECOMMENDED THERAPEUTIC PROCEDURES TO BE CARRIED OUT: ____________________

DIETARY RECOMMENDATION: ____________________

NEXT PHYSICAL OR FOLLOW-UP: ____________________ **ATTENDING VETERINARIAN:** ____________________

125M—2-69—IVES

Courtesy of Hill's Division Riviana Foods.

sonality or habits you have observed. The physical exam will take more time then your usual "check-up," and you may or may not be asked to be present during the entire examination. The laboratory work can take one to several days for completion, depending on whether it is done in the clinic lab or sent to an outside laboratory.

When all the information and results are put together and assessed by your veterinarian, you will be asked to come in to discuss them and any problems which may have been detected. If you've been giving your dog the proper care he deserves, you may be one of the fortunate ones to receive an "in good health—no detectable disorders" report. I fail to understand those dog owners who, upon receiving such good news, are disappointed and feel they have spent their money on "nothing." How can a report telling you that your aging dog is in good health and free of disease be thought of as "nothing?"

With the information this examination will provide each year, you and your family veterinarian together can keep your dog healthy and active during his extended lifetime. If you are not already familiar with your doctor's preventive medicine program, ask him about it during your next visit, which I hope will not have to wait until your dog is sick.

Sex and the Aging Dog

For ages Western society has tried to relegate older people to a sexually inactive life simply because they are old. Certainly there is no basis in nature for this attitude. All around us, animals of diverse types and sizes continue to be sexually active throughout their lives.

Many pet female dogs will already have had an ovariohysterectomy performed when they were young. But for those of you whose dogs are still intact, please read on. The normal estrus cycle (heat) of the bitch lasts twenty-one days, occurring every five to six months except in the giant breeds, which may cycle every eight to ten months. The vulva will swell, become inflamed, and there will be some amount of bleeding during almost the entire three-week period. She will be most receptive at this time to the attentions of male dogs and occasionally other female dogs. Keep her under control so that she doesn't become impregnated inadvertently. Should such a mismating take place, see your veterinarian immediately for an injection which often will prevent conception (see Mismating, page 121).

It is strongly recommended that bitches more than eight years old not be bred, unless there are truly urgent reasons for so doing. The physical and emotional stresses of pregnancy and delivery are considerable even for a younger dog. For the aging dog they can precipitate serious episodes of otherwise controlled disorders. The continuously enlarging pregnant uterus pushes all other abdominal organs out of its way. Pressure is applied to the stomach and intestines, often interfering with proper digestion and movement of food through these organs. The stomach is also forced forward against the diaphragm, thereby reducing the size of the chest cavity, making it more difficult for the lungs to fully expand and for the dog to breathe. Such pressures could change a latent heart or lung problem into an acute, life-threatening episode.

Obviously, if you have a valuable breeding bitch, you may wish to continue her productive years beyond eight. If you truly value her health and life as an individual dog, not just as a puppy-producing machine, she should have a complete geriatric physical exam and lab workup, as described further on, *before* each breeding.

OK, you've decided you're not going to breed her, but you live in the suburbs or on a farm, and your dog runs loose all the time. You can't suddenly lock her up for three weeks, twice a year—well, you can but you'd rather not. How to keep her from being impregnated by the local male dogs? There are at least two alternatives. In the early seventies, a so-called IUD—intra-uterine device—was developed for female dogs. It actually is placed only in the vagina, but IUD is a popular term so we're stuck with it. The device is made of an inert plastic material which has to be fitted to the individual bitch. Correctly and carefully placed by your family veterinarian at the beginning of the heat period, these devices quite effectively prevent male dogs from successfully copulating. When her period is over, the device is removed. As with any IUD, there are rare occurrences of irritation or infection, but these are usually the result of improper placement rather than the fault of the device itself.

For more than a decade, dog owners in Great Britain have been able to give their unspayed bitches a "pseudo-pill," which is now available in the United States. Unlike the "pill" for women, which prevents conception after copulation, the canine form of pill delays or prevents the heat cycle, so the bitch is unreceptive and uninteresting to the male. To be maximally effective, it must be started during a specific three-day-period at the beginning of the heat cycle and will postpone estrus for six to nine months. If begun before or after those three days, the effectiveness varies and will last a much shorter time. For the present, the drug is not recommended to be used for more than two consecutive heat periods. Every third estrus should be allowed to take place naturally. Perhaps in a decade or less, it will be cleared for use on every heat cycle, but even with its current limitation you can still obtain a fifteen to eighteen month respite from the annoyance and headaches of having a bitch in heat.

Several other chemical methods of preventing heat are under study at this time, including one which is incorporated into a commercial food, and another which implants the male hormone, testosterone, under the skin. Both are purported to have few undesirable side effects, and the hormone implant is said to last for up to two years. Hopefully, further research will soon produce methods which are completely safe and effective in the geriatric bitch.

A third alternative to consider is to have an ovariohysterectomy performed on your bitch. Many pros and cons can be heard on this subject. There seems to be significantly more objection to such an operation from women than from men. I suppose they unconsciously associate such an operation with how they would feel undergoing such surgery themselves. Even though they know that their dog will not experience the psychological problems encountered by some women, they are still reluctant. In favor of an OVH is the fact that once the uterus and ovaries are removed, your bitch cannot develop the very common uterine infection known as pyometra. The operation also reduces the chances of her getting breast tumors and, of course, precludes her coming into heat anymore. As long as your bitch is in good health, there is no greater surgical or anesthetic risk than if she were younger. Even for those with some degree of kidney or cardiovascular disease, the risk is not undue, what with today's newer and safer anesthetics. However, this obviously varies with each individual and you should follow the advice of your family veterinarian as to whether or not your geriatric bitch should have an ovariohysterectomy done.

For the aging male dog, sex does not pose quite such a problem. He can probably engage in an active sex life with safety well into advanced age. This is not intended to sound chauvinistic. It's simply that a male dog doesn't have to carry a family of puppies around in his body for nine weeks! Even so, he does have to be careful as he gets older. The act of copulation puts considerable strain on the hip and stifle joints, the vertebrae of the lower back, and many muscle groups. Arthritic joints, intervertebral disc disease, or weakening muscles may not only preclude successful copulation, but may be further injured by attempts to mate. It is important that you carefully supervise such matings to avoid any injuries, rather than just allowing the two dogs to run loose in the backyard.

The side effects of castrating an adult male dog can be quite diverse and extensive, ranging from rapid obesity to chronic lethargy and a physical femininization. Such surgery is rarely done except for medical reasons, such as tumor removal and prostate enlargement, or severe behavioral problems, such as viciousness which cannot be controlled by effective training. Recently many humane associations have insisted on the castration of all male dogs adopted from them. There are fewer and less extensive side effects to the operation when it is done on a young dog. Fortunately, not many aged dogs are likely to find their way into animal shelters.

There is no known medical need for a dog to engage in sexual activity. Despite popular misconceptions to the contrary (excuse the unintended pun), breeding does not cure false pregnancy, make a dog temperamentally better to be with children or, as I was recently told by a well-meaning new client who uses her male dog at stud once every three months, "it helps to keep him young looking."

Stress

It has been said several times that aging dogs are less adaptable to, and more adversely affected by, stress and change. Yet so many dog owners don't take this into consideration when making plans involving their geriatric dog. For years you and your dog enjoyed those races through the woods or around the playground. You may still enjoy it now, but your older dog possibly finds it difficult to keep up with you. What used to be lots of fun may now make her a bit grouchy and force her to breathe abnormally hard. You've just redecorated the house, and what used to be your dog's favorite spot to relax in, is now occupied by a piece of furniture. Your dog becomes restless, temperamental, may even urinate or defecate in the house or right on that piece of furniture, and you can't understand why.

It isn't necessary to baby or spoil a dog just because she is aging. In fact, this should be carefully avoided, as it is a trap into which many dog owners readily fall. You should encourage your older dog to take part in family life as always, but you must be alert to avoid undue stresses or unnecessary changes. That piece of new furniture doesn't *have to* stand on the exact spot where she has snoozed for more than ten years. In her mind that spot is her personal territory. Even in her youth such a loss would have been upsetting, but she'd soon find another acceptable location. The older dog finds it more difficult to adjust and can develop undesirable behavior as a result.

A dog is both a dependent and an independent animal in her relationship with you. In youth she will follow your every footstep even to the point of getting underfoot. Her greatest joy is to be with you everywhere, and there are few times she wants to be by herself. As she grows older, however, this will often change, and she may seek solitude much more of the time. She loves you still but, depending on her physical state, she just prefers to be by herself. She will play with you and be your companion, but don't expect necessarily the same kind of response you got from her when she was a lot younger.

Take care not to "kill her with kindness" by offering what you consider tasty morsels of human food—the leftover hors d'oeuvre, the caviar, the ice cream, the bacon, or the liver pâté. Such sudden changes in diet can produce serious stomach and intestinal upset, resulting in profuse vomiting or diarrhea. It may also encourage your dog to refuse her normal food and hold out for the "goodies." In time this can cause severe nutritional imbalances. Even if these problems don't arise, lots of goodies will almost surely lead to that bugaboo of "the good life"—obesity—which, as you have already read, can result in a shorter life.

There will frequently be times when you cannot take your dog with you—vacation, business out of town, health regulations—and you must leave her behind. Normally, any good boarding kennel would be the answer. For the older dog, accustomed to a routine of living, activity, and diet, there could be problems. Be sure that the floor of the kennel is not cold stone or concrete which can create difficulties for aging joints and weakening muscles. Wood, vinyl, or some other warm surface is preferable. And send along a familiar towel or blanket for her to lie on. Her own food and water dishes will also help her adjust to the strange surroundings. And be sure to provide enough of her regular diet to last the entire stay. A sudden change to the kennel's diet, no matter how good it may be, is very likely to cause diarrhea, vomiting, or even worse, complete refusal to eat.

Your geriatric dog may now be accustomed to being taken or let out quite a few times a day to urinate and defecate. The two- or three-time-a-day routine of most kennels can result in harmful retention of urine and feces or else their elimination right in the kennel, causing soiling of your dog's haircoat and skin.

Many boarding kennels prefer you not to send personal belongings with your dog, as they may get lost, require special cleaning and care, and so on. They also have fairly set daily routines and can be quite reluctant to change them. Nevertheless, there are good kennels in most areas that understand the special problems of boarding an older dog and that will cater to her special needs. In many cases there is no extra charge, while in others the additional cost is well worth it, in terms of your dog's health and comfort. Whenever you must board your dog, try to plan well in advance and make a definite reservation. Visit the kennel, and discuss your dog's special needs. If they seem understanding and cooperative, you're in the right place. But if your request for special care is met with a frown, head for the nearest door and look elsewhere. Friends who have older dogs may be able to recommend a kennel they used and were pleased with.

You will surely want to take your dog with you on some of your travels. As long as her overall health is good, there should be no serious obstacles. However, if she has a cardiovascular problem or an advanced musculoskeletal disorder such as arthritis, there is some question as to whether she should be subjected to the stresses of travel, be it by plane, train, or car. Your family veterinarian will be able to advise you whether or not to take her and, if yes, recommend specific precautionary measures to make the trip a safe one for your dog. Any vaccinations *required* for travel should be given at least one month before your trip so she'll have time to get over any possible reactions.

For a dog who is in general good health, the following suggestions will help make travel less stressful and more enjoyable.

By Car

- Make frequent stops, to allow your dog to stretch stiff legs as well as urinate and defecate, and to offer tiny amounts of water.
- Take enough of her regular diet with you, unless you are *sure* you can obtain it en route.
- Feed at your dog's regular feeding times but preferably in early morning and after the trip. If only once a day, it should be at least one hour after you finish driving for the day.
- If possible, feed outside of, rather than in, the car.
- Don't start driving again for at least two hours after feeding.
- Don't let your dog lie on the floor of the front seat. Engine and exhaust fumes accumulate most at that spot. Either the floor of the back seat or, if your dog is small enough, *on* the front or back seat is safer.
- Don't let her stand on her back legs or stick her head out of an open window. Any sudden change in the car's direction or speed can throw her off balance.
- When you stop for the night, walk her *slowly* for ten to fifteen minutes.
- Make certain, in advance, that your motel or hotel will allow dogs in your room, not just in a nearby kennel.
- Never leave your dog alone in the car, even for a few minutes.

By Plane

- Try to take your dog in the cabin with you. If small enough, most airlines will allow one dog in the cabin on each flight. Should she have to go as freight, be certain that the cargo area is fully pressurized and supplied with oxygen. Verify this when you make your reservation and keep on verifying it, especially when you check in at the airport. Sometimes a last-minute change in planes is necessary due to equipment problems, the substitute plane's cargo area may not be pressurized, and the airline personnel, busy as they always are, may just forget that a live dog is to be on that flight. So ask again when you are checking in!

• Don't feed your dog for two to four hours before the flight and not at all during the flight.

• As soon as you land, please claim your dog. Your luggage won't get sick sitting in a wet or drafty cargo area, but your dog will.

By Train

• It is probably best not to feed your dog at all during a train ride. In today's age of driving and flying, most train trips are short enough that your dog would not be made unduly hungry or thirsty.

• Get a parlor car, if at all possible, so you can keep your dog with you. Otherwise she will have to ride in a kennel in the baggage car, certainly a far more stressful situation.

The use of tranquilizers and motion sickness pills can be potentially hazardous for older dogs. They should never be given except on the advice and prescription of your veterinarian.

Personality Changes

Your dog's personality is a very subjective topic. Only you can perceive it for what it truly is. Actions and reactions by your dog to strangers, friends, and your veterinarian are usually characterized only by the stimulus of the immediate situation and not by her natural and normal personality.

As your dog's stress tolerance diminishes, her former interest in roughhousing with you may also be reduced. She may even resent your attempts at such play and respond with a warning growl which, if not respected, may lead to self-protective biting. Punishment under such circumstance could stimulate a continually aggressive state. It is also important you keep in mind that changes in personality, even in some of the extreme forms, are not synonymous with senility as that term is used when applied to people. *True senility is quite rare in dogs.*

Your older dog's need for your companionship may take either of two directions. On the one hand, she may seek an increasing amount of privacy or seclusion, not wanting to be within sight or sound of you for long periods of time other than for feeding or controlled outdoor activity. Respect her emotional needs and do not force yourself on her. Rather, be sensitive to those shorter periods when she does seek your company, respond with love and kindness, and find a way you can be satisfied and happy with this more aloof relationship.

On the other hand, your dog can become the exact opposite, seeking to be closer to you more and more of the time, not wanting to be left by herself. She may even *demand* your attention, crying, barking, or becoming destructive in order to get it and perhaps becoming aggressive toward any person she thinks is taking you away from her.

Both of these are extremes of their behavior genre. Fortunately, the personality of most aging dogs changes considerably less, whichever direction such changes may take. Within reason, indulge these common emotional needs of aging. Extremes should not be tolerated, however, and should prompt you to have your dog examined by your veterinarian. Many times he will find health problems causing the altered behavior. Painful, infected teeth, kidney or heart disease, tumors, or arthritic joints; all can produce adverse personality changes. Many of these can be corrected or improved, and with them the undesirable behavior. Should the examination rule out physiological reasons for such personality changes, behavioral modification therapy may be advised.

Chronic Neglect

Just as proper veterinary care cannot guarantee long life, it is also sometimes possible for a dog to live quite long with very little or no such care, but if I were a dog I certainly wouldn't want to count on it. I remember four dogs in particular, each of whom lived to be fifteen or more years old.

Bootey had not been to a doctor since she was ten. This shepherd had never been sick a day in her life, according to the owner, yet was presented to me in acute congestive heart failure and died during the examination.

Sidney hadn't seen a veterinarian for eight years. The owner couldn't understand why this terrier's teeth were rotting out, his heart and kidneys were diseased and he had difficulty walking. "Well, he's lived this long without veterinary treatment. I'm sure he'll keep on doing OK without your help" said the owner, and left with Sidney under his arm.

Ginger, another shepherd, had not been to a veterinarian since she had been a *puppy* and was a walking textbook of geriatric disorders—congestive heart failure, infected uterus, several breast tumors, kidney failure, lung tumors, and almost total blindness from glaucoma. The owner, herself quite elderly, said she didn't want Ginger to outlive her and therefore would not start any treatments. I'm sorry to say Ginger indeed did not outlive her owner or even see the summer that followed her springtime exam.

And then there was Doc, a Kerry blue terrier, whose teeth had been bad for four years but whose owner kept putting off having them cleaned. When Doc developed a serious kidney infection from them, he had the dog euthanized.

Yes, in spite of such chronic neglect by some owners, it appears that compassionate and benevolent "Doctor Nature" occasionally sees fit to keep such dogs alive for many years.

2
When Your Dog Is Sick

You and your dog have been together many years—five, ten, perhaps fifteen—and have shared many good and bad times. When you were a child, you could tell your parents if something hurt or was not well with you. Even as an infant you could at least cry to indicate something was amiss. Alas, our canine pets cannot do either. Besides, a dog's pain threshhold seems to be considerably higher than that of humans, and they will not whimper or cry until the discomfort is quite severe. It is therefore necessary that you know so well what is normal for *your* dog, any changes will be quickly detected.

How to Tell If Your Mature Dog Is Sick

Now I think we can both agree that no one knows your dog's normal habits and patterns better than you! However, because of this very fact, you may allow yourself to become less observant of your dog, so that slight or subtle changes from the normal may go unnoticed until they are grossly abnormal and appear to have "come up overnight." One good way to avoid this is to develop the following habits of observation.

• On first greeting your dog in the morning, stop what you are doing, and watch her for one full minute, allowing her to move about as she wishes.

• During the morning and evening outdoor activity, observe her for ten seconds as she moves up or down stairs, on and off a curbing, porch, etc. Let her walk a short distance ahead of you and watch her body movements for ten seconds.

• Once a day observe the first twenty seconds of eating a meal, a full twenty seconds during sleep, a complete urination, and a complete bowel movement.

Many subtle variations from your dog's normal patterns will be noticed by doing this, even though you are not looking for specifics. In addition, unconsciously noticed changes will register on your brain and, during the giving of the medical history at your veterinarian's clinic, they will come into your conscious memory. If gross abnormalities are seen, resist the urge to get upset and excited. Try to objectively watch those abnormalities, so you will be able to describe accurately what has occurred.

Like all habits—and this observation pattern should become a habit—it will take practice at first, but it will eventually occupy only a total of four to six minutes spread out over your waking day. Surely you can make that little bit of time available to protect the health of someone who brings you so much pleasure and happiness.

Most symptoms of illness are vague, general, nonspecific, or all three. A single symptom, by itself, is often meaningless, at best, and misleading at worst. There are so-called pathognomonic symptoms which supposedly, in and of themselves, indicate a specific illness or disease. While such symptoms do exist, they are few and far between.

I have divided the following signs and symptoms into three groups. The first contains those which, if they happen only once or occasionally—*not repeatedly*—during a twenty-four-hour period, you can probably dismiss as nothing to be worried about. That is, providing they are not recurring every day or two! The second group lists those signs and symptoms which usually mean that something is wrong with your dog, although perhaps nothing serious, and should be brought to the attention of your veterinarian. The last group includes those signs and symptoms which indicate serious or potentially serious disorders and should be considered as true danger signals warranting your prompt action.

Group 1	Vomiting food without blood	Loss of appetite
	Diarrhea without blood	Sneezing
	Very hard stool or none at all	Loss of pep
	Coughing	Lethargy
Group 2	Tires easily and frequently	Inflamed or heavily discharging eyes
	Fever	Loss of muscle mass or tone
	Sudden increase in appetite	Stiffness in gait
	Increase or decrease in urination	Reluctance to walk or jump
	Increase in water intake	Lameness
	Unaccounted for loss or gain in weight—gradual or sudden	
	Diarrhea with blood	
Group 3	Prolonged rapid or difficult breathing	Walking into objects
	Change in tongue color—bright red, pale or bluish-purple	Sudden collapse, *even briefly*
	Repeated vomiting with blood	Inability to walk or jump
	Straining to defecate	Seizures, fits, or convulsions
	Straining to urinate	
	Dizziness	

Visiting Your Veterinarian

WHEN TO GO AND WHEN NOT TO GO

You've just awakened from a delightful night's sleep and, with the sun coming up brightly, it's surely going to be a beautiful day. Rover runs in to greet you and, seeing the bright sun, agrees with your prediction for the day. He romps playfully with you, tugging at your slippers as if to say—come on, I'm hungry, aren't you? His food prepared, you give it to him in his favorite bowl. In no time flat, the food has disappeared, Rover is licking his chops and wagging his tail in contentment. You sit down to your own breakfast as Rover lies down happily where he can savor the joy of just watching you. Breakfast over, you are relishing that last bit of coffee when Rover begins to groan. Suddenly he sits up, retches, gags, and proceeds to vomit up all the food he has just eaten. As soon as he finishes throwing up, however, he calmly goes off to another room to play with his favorite rawhide toy, acting as if nothing unusual had happened.

Rover is not likely to be really sick. He may have eaten too fast, drank too much water after eating, the food might have been too hot or too cold, or perhaps the dish contained traces of left over food from the night before which had started to spoil. Your dog is acting quite normal now and you do *not* have to rush off to your veterinarian or even call him. Just take away all food and water for several hours and let him rest. *Exception*—if your dog is a cardiac or diabetic patient, has a history of urinary infection, kidney or liver disease, or is known to frequently swallow foreign material, call your veterinarian!

Let's go back to that beautiful morning again. This time Rover doesn't run in to greet you. You find him in another room, alert and bright but seemingly not in the mood for romping. The sounds and aromas of your preparing his food, which normally would bring him racing in, don't interest him. When you call to him, he comes and, to make you happy, eats some of the food but reluctantly. Then he goes back to where you first found him and lies down with a sad look in his eyes. These events should start a red flag waving inside your head! "Something is wrong. I don't know if it's serious but I better watch Rover carefully." Immediately remove all food and water. If you can observe him for two or three hours, and he shows no obvious improvement, get on the phone to your veterinarian. But you have to go off to work. A visit home at lunchtime, or having a neighbor look in on him, will put your mind at ease. If he's improved, great! If he is worse you still have time to get your dog to a veterinarian the same day.

Once more, let's go back to that seemingly beautiful morning. As before, Rover has eaten reluctantly, looks sick, and lies down with a woe-begotten look to him. This time he vomits, not only the food he ate, but some foul-smelling brownish-black liquid as well. He continues to retch, bringing up more brown fluid followed by a deep yellow liquid flecked with dark red spots and streaks. Oh-Oh, you just know that must be blood. And you're probably right. First take away all food and water, as Rover may try to eat or drink again and just vomit some more. Second, phone your veterinarian and arrange for him to see your dog.

As you can readily see, there are times when it is not necessary to rush your dog in for medical treatment, and other times when your dog's life may depend upon your prompt action. It is not always as relatively easy to decide what to do as in the three vignettes just presented. A good general rule of thumb that I advise my clients to use is—*if in doubt, phone me.* I would rather be a little disturbed by your overzealousness than fighting mad by your neglect of your dog. It is so easy in an older dog for those comparatively simple problems to become major ones by "hoping the symptoms will go away by tomorrow."

In the section How to Tell If Your Mature Dog Is Sick, I briefly divided a few signs and symptoms into three groups of increasing urgency. Now I would like to classify them and others into two groups—*Go* to your veterinarian and *Don't Go* to your veterinarian. Obviously I cannot list all possible symptoms of disorders. I have tried to include those which are especially important in the geriatric dog. Signs which are more likely seen in young dogs have been excluded, as have those found in any-age dog which are readily apparent, such as fleas, fractures, burns, hives, and so on. It should also be clear, from these two groups, that there are fewer times when you probably don't have to go to your veterinarian than when you definitely should go. The aging dog has fewer minor problems amenable to home treatment by you. Most geriatric problems are major ones or will rapidly become major if not properly treated.

Go means just that—no ifs, ands, or buts! However, *Don't Go* applies only if symptoms do not continue for more than twelve to twenty-four hours, do not get worse, or do not repeat every two or three days. Once again, an exact dividing line cannot be drawn. If in doubt, phone your doctor.

Don't Go

Appetite decreased during hot or humid weather
Appetite, temporary loss

Bowel movement sluggish
Bowel movement softer than usual, but formed
Coughing, occasional
Cuts or abrasions if superficial or minor
Diarrhea without visible blood
Discharge, slight, from otherwise clear eyes
Grass eating and resultant vomiting
Nose, hot or dry
Pep, temporary loss
Scratching, occasional
Shivering, occasional
Sneezing, occasional
Thirst increased during hot or humid weather
Urination increased during hot or humid weather
Vomiting food without visible blood

Go

Abdomen distended, other than obesity
Appetite, sudden increase
Blood from anywhere except minor cuts
Breath, foul-smelling
Breathing, rapid or difficult
Collapsing, no matter how briefly
Conjunctiva pale
Conjunctiva yellowish in color
Convulsions, fits, seizures
Coughing, repeated, especially if at night
Diarrhea with visible blood
Dizziness
Eyes cloudy or heavily discharging
Eyes sunken into their sockets
Fever higher than 103 °F (39.4 °C)
Gagging for more than one day
Gait, abnormal
Gums, pale
Gums, yellowish in color
Hair, excessive loss
Head shaking, frequent

Head, tilted or held down a lot
Hearing loss
Lameness
Licking or biting at hind quarters
Muscles, loss of mass or tone
Obesity
Odor, abnormal, from ears, mouth, anus, vulva, or skin
Pain anywhere
Paralysis
Pupils widely dilated or tightly constricted
Pus discharge from ear, vulva, or anus
Reluctance to walk or jump
Salivation, unaccounted for
Scratching, prolonged or continual
Scooting on anus
Skin, dry or waxy to the touch
Skin, inflamed or reddened with or without scratching or chewing
Sneezing, repeated, especially if with blood
Straining to defecate
Straining to urinate
Swallowing with difficulty
Swellings anywhere on body which persist more than twenty-four hours
Teeth, discolored, loose, or foul-smelling
Temperature *lower* than 100 °F (37.8 °C)
Tircs casily
Tongue, bluish, gray, very red, or pale
Urination, increase or decrease during *normal* weather.
Vision loss
Vomiting brown, black, or bloody fluid
Walking into objects
Water intake, increase or decrease during *normal* weather
Weakness or unsteadiness
Weight loss or increase, gradual or sudden

Having determined that you should go, you are now phoning your family veterinarian to arrange for him to see your dog. In most clinics and hospitals, you will speak with the receptionist.

Explain clearly what has happened and whether or not *you* feel it is urgent. Many receptionists today have had some medical training or have been trained by their employer to be able to determine what is really an emergency and also to give temporary advice while arranging your visit to the doctor. However, you may feel that the condition warrants an earlier visit than the one offered or more specific temporary advice. Don't hesitate to ask to speak with the doctor. It is rare, in private practice, that a veterinarian will not come to the phone, although this sometimes does occur in large institutional practices. Keep in mind that if he is with a patient, the doctor may not be able to speak with you immediately, but the receptionist will ask him to return your call promptly and give you an approximate time range within which he will do so. When he does, again give him an accurate, but brief, history. Remember, he probably has another patient waiting for him, but do not assume that the receptionist explained everything to him. He will then reschedule your appointment, if he feels it is necessary and give you as much temporary advice as you need.

Today most veterinarians conduct their practice on an appointment system. This allows them to plan enough time for each patient to be properly examined. If you arrive late, there will be less time available to examine your dog, or else the next patient, who is on time, will have to be kept waiting. Of course there are extenuating circumstances, so if it looks like you're going to be late, phone ahead. It is also possible that the doctor will be late for your appointment due to an emergency. Appointment systems notwithstanding, emergencies are taken immediately, and clients with appointments are asked to be understanding and considerate. After all, that dog just brought in having a convulsion or the one in congestive heart failure and looking very blue could have been your dog, and you surely wouldn't want to have to wait for an appointment to have his life saved!

HOW TO GIVE A GOOD HISTORY

Okay! Your appointment time has arrived, and you are now in the consultation or examining room with your dog. Either the doctor or a trained assistant (receptionist, technician, nurse) will take the history. In a very busy practice, it is not always possible for the doctor to do this herself, so don't be upset or feel slighted that your dog's history is being taken by a nonveterinarian. These assistants are carefully trained to elicit an accurate history from you, *but you must, of course, cooperate*.

You may wonder why I added those last six words. It's obvious that the owner must cooperate, you are saying to yourself. Well, obvious or not, there are owners who, not only do not cooperate, but actually attempt to mislead or confuse the persons trying to help their dog. Much of this stems from conscious or subconscious guilt feelings. "I saw that lump two months ago and thought it would go away but now it's three times bigger. I can't admit that, so I'll say it just appeared a few days ago." Or this one? "I woke up this morning to find my aged dog staggering around and falling down once in a while. We had a real blast of a party last night and . . . well . . . we gave her some liquor. I know that wasn't too smart, but she did like it, and it was funny to watch her. Then I think someone gave her uppers . . . or were they downers . . . or something. Heck, I can't tell all that to the doctor . . . it might get me into trouble. The dog is old anyway, so I'll suggest she had a stroke or heart attack. Maybe the doctor won't discover the real cause." Sound crazy, fantastic, hard to believe? Both situations actually did occur, and there is hardly a veterinarian who hasn't been confronted with similar ones.

And what about the client who, when questioned about his dog, answers with "You're the doctor! Why are you asking me? I'm paying you to find out!"

Your veterinarian is in clinical companion animal practice to help your dog, but she can accomplish this only through you. Your dog cannot refute your statements directly, although the examination findings may cast serious doubt on their accuracy. A factual, accurate history is the essential foundation of a proper examination and correct diagnosis and, in emergencies, can save great amounts of time. Some doctors may ask you to give the history in your own words and sequence, as you see it. Others may ask you detailed and very specific questions, keeping you on the track and not allowing you to wander from the immediate problem. Most will use a combination of both methods. If the assistant is taking the history, he has been trained to record everything in confidence, and you should speak freely. However, if there is something in the history which you feel you cannot discuss with the assistant, tell him so. He will make a note of it to the doctor who will then discuss it with you.

During the course of the examination, additional history may be requested by the doctor, or some questions repeated for clarification. Be as accurate as you can, but under no circumstances state as a fact something you are only guessing at. If you aren't sure, say so. If you don't know at all, say so. It is better to give a few bits of reliable information than a plethora of guesses and misinformation.

Questions you might be asked include: Have there been any major illnesses previously? Has there been any coughing, sneezing, vomiting, diarrhea? If yes, for how long—a day, several weeks, longer? Is there blood in the vomitus or diarrhea? Is the blood bright red or pink or very dark red or black? Is the urine normal in color, and has the frequency or amount changed in any way? Does your dog strain before, during, or after urinating? Does the cough occur more at night than during the day? When your dog is active or at rest or during sleep? Does it wake the dog up at night? Does the lameness improve, get worse, or stay the same when your dog gets up from sleep and has walked around for a while? Does he hold the leg up and hop on three legs, or does he touch it lightly to the ground, or perhaps he drags it behind him? Does the lameness shift from one leg to another? Is it worse during periods of cold or high humidity?

And so the medical sleuthing begins. Like a detective, your veterinarian will collect facts from you, from the physical exam of your dog, and from diagnostic tests. They will be analyzed, compared, and combined in order to arrive at a diagnosis.

Having decided to take your dog to whichever veterinarian you are now talking to, have confidence in her and trust her. Remember, her primary goal is to help you and your dog. If you do not honestly believe that, you had best find another veterinarian for your dog!

In the event you have recently moved to a new area or city or, for some other reason, you have changed veterinarians, there will be an additional type of history your new doctor will need. She will ask you about all previous major and minor illnesses your mature dog has had as well as prior immunizations. Try to recall these to the best of your ability. Of course, if you've kept a personal medical diary on your dog, as so many dog owners are doing today, it will be much simpler. You probably will be asked to contact your former veterinarian—whether she is down the block or across the country—and request that your dog's complete medical history be sent to your new doctor. Often a phone call is all that is needed, but many veterinarians do ask that such a request, for what is really very personal information, be made in writing. This information is important in diagnosing any dog, but is especially so in the aging dog, as former illnesses very often have a direct bearing on geriatric problems.

Sometimes I've had a client say, when asked to request such records, "I'd rather Dr. so-and-so didn't know I've changed veterinarians" or "I've come for a second opinion without Dr. so-and-so's knowledge. I'd be embarrassed to tell him now." Every veterinarian knows, and should accept the fact, that clients will change doctors for a wide variety of reasons, all of which seem valid to the client. It is your right and privilege to choose whichever doctor you wish. It is also your prerogative to obtain a second opinion (see The Diagnosis), but common courtesy should prompt you to advise your doctor of your intention to do so. Yes, you may be embarrassed if you haven't told him, but the records will be made available. Your veterinarian, I am sure, is able to put the welfare of his former patient ahead of any real or imagined slight to his ego.

THE DIAGNOSIS

The history, physical exam, and diagnostic tests having been analyzed and compared, your veterinarian will arrive at some form of diagnosis. Ideally, it should be a *definitive* diagnosis—"your dog has this specific illness." Unfortunately, this is not always possible, and it is considerably more difficult to do in older patients. Your dog is a living being undergoing continual physiological change, so that diagnoses may not be clearly black and white but rather varying shades of gray. In such cases, it may only be possible to give a *provisional* diagnosis. This means all facts seem to point toward a particular problem but not clearly so. Additional tests or a trial period of certain medications may be needed to see what change, if any, they produce in the illness. In some of the more difficult to diagnose disorders, such as certain internal tumors, your veterinarian may initially be able to offer only a group of *differential* diagnoses. It is then necessary to pursue each one until a provisional, and eventually, a definitive diagnosis is arrived at. Until such time, he will have to treat your dog symptomatically; that is, treat the observed symptoms without knowing specifically what is causing them, until the definitive diagnosis is made. Occasionally the dog responds to such symptomatic therapy and gets well without a definitive diagnosis ever being reached.

A broken bone, infected ears, certain parasitic skin problems, bad teeth, heartworm disease—these are usually amenable to a definitive diagnosis. Failing vision, increased thirst and urination, chronic coughing, chronic vomiting or diarrhea, or rapid breathing frequently permits only a provisional diagnosis at first. A differential list of diagnoses may be all your veterinarian can give you on the first examination for many types of kidney and liver ailments, anemias, or immune, neurological or nutritional disorders.

You have just been given a definitive diagnosis. It will require some home treatment or perhaps a short period of hospitalization, and your dog will, in all likelihood, recover. You agree to have your veterinarian do this, and you go home confident that all will be well. On the other hand, that diagnosis may indicate the need for a major operation, a long hospitalization, the use of potentially dangerous medications, incurring a large expense, or your commitment to prolonged or continuing aftercare. You have confidence in your veterinarian and, after a thorough discussion of what will be done, agree to go ahead. Or, even though you have confidence, because of the serious nature of what is involved, you would like a second opinion.

As stated previously, it is your right and privilege to request a second opinion, and every veterinarian understands that. Do not hesitate to tell the doctor of your wishes. He will appreciate your genuine concern and help you find a consultant. I usually suggest the names of at least two or three other veterinarians whom I feel are especially competent in the particular problem involved. They are doctors whom I will frequently consult with, myself, when I have a difficult diagnostic problem. The client then selects one and arranges for the appointment. If you would rather choose a doctor other than those recommended, that is again your right, and your veterinarian will understand. When you go to the consultant, it is to your dog's advantage to tell him that you have come for a second opinion and that you have already been elsewhere. If you request them, your first doctor will send copies of his findings, laboratory results, and radiographs to your consulting veterinarian.

Following his examination, if the consultant agrees with your original doctor's diagnosis, he should refer you back for follow-up, and all records will be returned. If you have valid reasons why you do not wish to return and want the consultant to treat your dog, you should so notify the first doctor, so he knows that your dog's illness is being cared for. In the event the consultant does not confirm the diagnosis or agree with the proposed course of therapy, he will so advise the referring doctor. You again have the option of choosing who will treat your dog. If your pet has been under the care of one veterinarian for a number of years, it is to your dog's advantage to be treated by that doctor, since he knows your dog's medical history in detail, better than anyone else. Don't be surprised, however, if your veterinarian himself recommends that the consultant follow through with therapy, if he feels that would be better for your dog.

I am reminded in a way of Rags, an eleven-year-old terrier mix, whose veterinarian of at least the last eight of those years had diagnosed two very small breast tumors. Surgical removal and an ovariohysterectomy were advised. Rags' owner didn't like what she heard and took her to another doctor who, unknown to the owner, no longer included surgery in his practice. The second doctor said there were no tumors, and Rags should not be spayed. The owner was happy but surprised, and more than a bit confused. A friend recommended she bring Rags to me. The breast tissue in question was very deeply imbedded and difficult to find but most certainly was abnormal. Suggesting that it be examined again in two to four weeks before deciding upon surgery, I otherwise concurred with the original veterinarian's assessment and recommendations, and referred Rags back to him. In less than three weeks, the astute doctor was able to show clearly the growing tumors to the owner. Surgery was authorized, and Rags made an uneventful recovery. The joyful owner called to tell me the tumors were malignant but had not spread anywhere. I heard from her again a couple of years ago when Rags was celebrating her seventeenth birthday. There had been no recurrences, and she was still going strong!

The decision as to who will treat your ailing dog has now been made. Although much discourse has already passed between you and the veterinarian, a thorough discussion about what will be done—at surgery, in the hospital, at home—and what results can reasonably be expected should now take place. No veterinarian can guarantee the results of *any* therapy, and you'd better start walking out of his office if he says he can. He should, however, be able to give you the reasonable likelihood of success—but not in percentages, unless he's a gambling man. He should explain to you in language you can understand—maybe you understand medicalese, maybe you don't—what types of treatments or surgery will be done, what additional diagnostic procedures might be needed, and what untoward problems could occur, such as side effects of medications.

While your veterinarian cannot take the time to give you a short course in the diagnosis and treatment of your dog's disorder, he will try to answer any questions not already covered in his explanation. He should also be able to give you an approximate idea of how long therapy will take, and for how long there might be follow-up care at home or follow-up visits to the clinic. At this time you should be sure to discuss the estimated cost of what will be done and make definite arrangements as to how these fees will be paid. Depending upon the nature of your dog's illness, there may be more than one possible course of treatment. Your doctor will explain each to you and either make a recommendation, let you choose the therapy, or both.

If Your Dog Needs Hospitalization

I don't know anyone who enjoys staying in a hospital even if it is for a minor ailment. There are strange sounds, strange odors, strange people, and a very different and highly organized daily routine. Though people may gripe about being hospitalized, most adjust fairly rapidly to the pattern without becoming depressed or it in any way affecting their ability to get well. In time, some few may even get to like their new environment.

In the veterinary clinic, it is a rare dog who complains about his hospital stay. Most adjust to the numerous changes within a day or two. Some canines, like those few people, really do enjoy the new environment, if they are not too seriously ill. They act almost as if they had forgotten their home and owner, although I'm sure that doesn't completely happen. I believe they simply accept the fact of their hospital stay and temporarily put other thoughts out of their mind. There are two general exceptions to this majority. The first is young puppies eight to twelve weeks old who are just establishing their canine-human social relationship. The second exception is the well-loved and deeply attached aged dog. For the senior citizens of the dog world, hospitalization is more likely to be emotionally distressing. The importance of avoiding stress for these dogs has been set forth earlier.

Your family veterinarian is keenly aware of the potentially adverse effects hospitalization may have on your older dog and will try to avoid it whenever it is medically possible. This will require your cooperation, as it may necessitate daily or even twice daily visits in order to treat your dog as an out-patient, depending on how sick he is. With diligence and teamwork, many such out-patients can be restored to good health without having to be separated from their accustomed environment for more than brief periods each day.

Sometimes, out-patient therapy does not produce satisfactory results for very long. At other times, the life-threatening nature of the illness or the type of treatments needed preclude therapy as an out-patient. Hospitalization becomes a necessity, but your veterinarian will do everything possible to reduce its stresses and possible negative effects. He might ask you to bring a favorite dish, blanket, or other object from home that will make the different environment seem a bit more familiar and reassuring. In many hospitals the care and treatment of your dog will be assigned to just one doctor and one veterinary attendant or nurse in order for your dog to become familiar and feel more secure with them. Too many different faces can be upsetting. The doctor and attendant will try to provide some of the love and affection your dog needs, as well as his medical requirements. Treatment and care will be more individualized for your aging dog and will absorb much more of the doctor's time.

The question of visiting your dog is a difficult one to answer. Almost all dogs are upset the first day away from their owners. To whatever extent he does adjust to the separation, a visit from you will end with a new parting and undo the adjustment he has made. For this reason many veterinary hospitals and clinics do not permit direct visiting. The marvels of modern technology, however, have provided a way for you to see your dog without him seeing you. Closed circuit television is to be found in many hospitals today, so you can observe your dog in a distant ward without upsetting him or any other patient in that ward. On rare occasions, a dog is truly distressed by hospitalization to such an extent that he "gives up the fight" and will not respond adequately to otherwise effective therapy. Under such circumstances your doctor will invite you to visit with your dog as often as is necessary to stimulate renewed response. Remember, though, your dog needs reassurance and confidence from you at such times, so please do your utmost to avoid tears, or any reaction other than a loving happy smile and voice, until after you have left the ward.

As soon as your dog's health has improved sufficiently to be *safely* treated as an out-patient, he will be discharged from the hospital. It is essential that you speak directly with the doctor at the time of discharge and get full, detailed instructions from him for your dog's proper care at home. I do not believe this vital responsibility can be left to a nurse or receptionist, no matter how well trained such a person might be. Unfortunately, the larger the hospital, the less likely you are to see the doctor, but do attempt to insist on it. Make certain you know how medications are to be administered and at what intervals, what to expect as a result of the medications, what possible side effects may occur and, perhaps most important, what signs should get you on the phone to the doctor.

If Your Dog Needs Surgery and Anesthesia

Until the late fifties and early sixties, the prospect for a successful outcome of many surgical procedures in older dogs was somewhat dubious. This was due in small part to the surgical techniques and materials employed at the time, but primarily to the types of anesthetics then available. Those anesthetics were often unpredictable, sometimes produced longer periods of anesthesia than were needed for the operation, and they had to be detoxified and eliminated largely by the liver and kidneys, organs which usually are already under stress in the older dog. These problems sometimes prompted many conscientious veterinarians to advise clients that "your dog is too old to anesthetize or be operated on." What they were really saying was that the risk from surgery and anesthesia was at least as great, or greater, than the risk from whatever was wrong with the dog.

Today that situation has radically changed. Anesthetizing a seriously ill geriatric patient is still in the high-risk category, but the chances of a successful outcome are tremendously improved. The new types of inhalation (gas) anesthetics give excellent control over the depth and time of anesthesia and allow for rapid recovery to a normal, conscious state. In addition, better equipment for their administration has made these, as well as some of the older, gas anesthetics much safer. Many of the newer and much safer injectable anesthetics can be used alone for general anesthesia or, in combination with some gas anesthetics, to provide "balanced anesthesia." And certainly, the ready availability of artificial respirators which can breathe for your dog has both increased the overall safety of anesthesia as well as permitted surgery within the chest cavity for some types of cardiac and lung disorders.

No dog should be considered "too old" for surgery or anesthesia if otherwise in reasonable health. The aging kidneys and liver still must detoxify much of the anesthetic, aging lungs can make inhalant anesthetics more difficult to control, and heart disease does increase the overall danger. There still is risk, but it is a calculated risk, usually weighted on the side of success.

In today's modern veterinary hospitals and clinics, surgery is done under conditions similar to those found in human hospitals. Everything is done to keep the surgical area sterile, which includes doctors scrubbing before surgery and wearing sterile cap, mask, and gown. All instruments, surgical drapes, and any piece of equipment that will come in contact with the patient is sterilized. The surgery is performed in a separate operating room, which is used only for sterile surgery. While each operating room will vary in the variety of equipment available, it will have whatever is needed for the particular operation being done. If your veterinarian's hospital is not equipped to perform a particular type of surgery, he will refer you to a colleague who does have the necessary equipment, or he may do the surgery himself but in his colleague's hospital.

Occasionally an operation requires more than one surgeon or a surgical team. If your doctor is the only veterinarian in his hospital, veterinarians from other hospitals and clinics will "scrub in" with him to assure the successful outcome of the operation.

Following surgery, your dog will be kept in a recovery ward where she will be carefully observed until fully recovered and back to normal. Oxygen and other emergency equipment will be available in the recovery area should any adverse postanesthetic problems arise, an uncommon but possible occurrence.

Postsurgical stays in the hospital are not as long today as in bygone years. Of course, the nature of the operation and your dog's overall state of health will dictate the length of her stay, but you will have her home just as soon as it is safe for her to be there.

Drugs—How to Use and Not Use Them

Modern drugs are surely a boon to the practice of veterinary medicine. They have helped save the lives of many critically ill dogs and restored countless others to normal health. Yet improperly used, they can not only fail in their intended function, but can actually create a more serious threat to your dog. An antibiotic given at haphazard and infrequent intervals can create a resistant strain of bacteria. A corticosteroid abruptly discontinued after long use can precipitate a dangerous adrenal gland hormone imbalance. A drug intended to be given four times a day may produce a dangerously high blood level if given, only twice a day, but at double the dose.

When your veterinarian dispenses or prescribes medication for your aging dog she should also give you the following information in addition to the dose and frequency. If she doesn't *do not hesitate to ask.*

- What is the medication expected to do?
- How soon can improvement be expected?
- How long should you wait if there is no change?
- How long should the medication be continued?
- Is the medicine to be stopped abruptly or is the dose to be reduced and how?
- Does the medicine need special storage? Away from light? Refrigeration? Must it be kept airtight?
- What possible side effects might be expected?

The dispensing label or prescription should carry specific directions for use, which should be followed explicitly. Is the medication to be given before or after or with food, or perhaps on an empty stomach which should remain empty for a specified time? Some medicines are inactivated by food, due to mechanical or chemical interference with their absorption from the stomach or small intestine.

If there is more than one type of medication, can they be given together, or is there a particular sequence of administration or time interval between them? Certain drugs interfere with each other when given together while others will intensify the reaction.

The directions say "three times daily." Does that mean morning, noon, and night or breakfast, lunch, and supper or every eight hours? The effective levels in the blood of some medications fall more rapidly than others and require administration at regular and specific time intervals.

The prescribed tablet is rather large and not too easy to administer twice a day. Will it be just as good to give a half-tablet four times a day? For some drugs the answer is yes. For others definitely not—by so doing you will render the drug ineffective.

And you most certainly will want to know when to start giving the drug—when you get home, later that day, the next morning, or only if certain symptoms appear?

Ask your veterinarian all pertinent questions before you leave the examining room! This is especially true if the prescription is to be filled outside of the veterinary hospital.

Many medications are available in different physical forms such as tablets, capsules, liquids, or powders, while others can be supplied in only one form. Having had your dog for many years, you may have developed greater skill at giving a tablet than a liquid or vice versa. It may be easier for you to apply ointment to an eye than to put in drops. Should you have such preferences, make your veterinarian aware of it. While any given drug may not be available in the form you prefer, your doctor will try to accommodate you when possible. In any case, ask your doctor to *show* you how to administer the medication, if you do not feel confident about how to do it. I will try to explain some methods of giving medicine, but no written description can be as effective as your seeing it done.

GIVING CAPSULES OR TABLETS

To start with, it is a rare dog who will eat a tablet or capsule placed in his food. Most will eat around it and leave the medication, carefully licked clean, at the bottom of the empty food dish. Of course, some powders and liquids are specifically made to be mixed with food and will usually be accepted by your dog, but tablets or capsules not intended to be used this way may lose some of their effectiveness when crushed into and mixed with food. In the aging dog, many medications have a critical effectiveness level, and a dose left in the food dish or spit out somewhere under a piece of furniture can radically alter that drug's action. For that reason I believe the best and surest way to give oral medication is to place it *directly* into your dog's mouth and make him swallow it. The following methods are outlined for a right-handed person. Southpaws will have to reverse the directions.

Have all the medications you are going to give ready before you call and position your dog. Don't start opening bottles or envelopes after she's there!

Set your dog in a sitting position with her head facing toward your right and her hind quarters to your left. Talk to her quietly and reassuringly. Place your left hand, palm down, over the top of her muzzle, and bring your fingers down, your thumb on the near side and the other four fingers on the far side of her mouth. Raise the head to a forty-five degree angle above the horizontal. Gently, but firmly, press the upper lips inward with your fingers, and as you continue to press inward, she will start to open her mouth. As long as you keep her lips between your fingers and her upper teeth, she will not close her mouth. If she did, she would have to bite her own lips—an unlikely event. With the mouth partially open, pick up the tablet or capsule in your right hand, holding it between thumb and forefinger. Using the middle finger of your right hand, take hold of the lower front teeth, *not* the lower lip, and pull the mouth open, wide enough to place all your fingers, and even your entire hand, into your dog's mouth. The more of your hand that is in her mouth the less she is able to close it.

Place the tablet or capsule as far back into the mouth as possible. Looking into the mouth you will note that your dog's tongue abruptly curves downward at the rear of her mouth. At that point, there is a small inverted V-shaped area on the midline which disappears around the downward curve of the tongue. Placement of the medication in the V-area will normally stimulate the swallowing reflex. Remove both hands quickly, gently hold the dog's mouth closed, and swallowing should take place. Some dogs will not swallow but will hold the medication in place until you release the mouth and will then spit it out. In that case keep the mouth closed, extend the head upward and gently stroke the throat. This will quite often stimulate swallowing. Should this not work let her spit it out, take a fresh tablet (the first will have become sticky and hard to manipulate), and try again. Don't be discouraged— practice *will* make perfect. By the way, be sure you place or push the capsule into the V-area. If you try to throw or drop it in, your dog will more than likely throw it right back out.

Some dogs will swallow a very small tablet if hidden in a "meatball" of food, but this is not always dependable. If it does work with your dog, be sure you use her normal food and deduct that amount from her regular meals.

GIVING LIQUID MEDICINES

Never give liquids by pouring them down the back of the throat. To do so almost assures that some of it will go into the windpipe and down into the lungs. The possibly resulting inhalation or aspiration pneumonia can be very difficult to treat.

Once again, set your dog in a sitting position facing to your right. Place your left thumb between the upper and lower lips where they come together to form the cheek and, with the thumb inside and index finger outside, pull the cheek slightly away from the teeth. This forms a pocket between the cheek and teeth. Please note that the mouth is *not* opened. Give the liquid with a dropper, spoon, narrow-mouthed bottle, or a dosing syringe, depending on the size of your dog and the amount of fluid to be given. Carefully place it into the cheek pocket and give the liquid in very small increments. By tipping the head up about thirty degrees above the horizontal, the fluid will run back into the pocket, flow between the back teeth, and stimulate the swallowing reflex. Be sure to allow a few seconds for your dog to swallow and breathe before you give more liquid. If a large amount must be given, let her rest every minute or two, releasing her lip but not letting her run off somewhere.

APPLYING EYE MEDICATION

Eye medications can sometimes be tricky to apply, especially if you have a terrier or other live-wire breed. Still with your dog facing to your right, separate the eyelids with the thumb and index fingers of your left hand as you steady her head with the rest of that hand. Take the tube of ointment in your right hand and rest the heel of that hand against your dog's face or muzzle. This way, if she moves her head suddenly, your right hand and the metal tube of ointment will move together with the head, and you won't end up poking her in the eye with the tube. Squeeze the tube so just a very small amount of ointment starts to ooze out and touch the ointment, not the tube, to the surface of the eyeball. If you flick your right wrist the ointment will generally stay on the eyeball. With your left thumb and forefinger, close the eyelids and very gently massage them for two or three seconds. The heat from the lids will melt the ointment and spread it all over the eye. Keep your dog occupied for a few minutes until she forgets about trying to paw at the eye.

When putting in eyedrops the procedure is similar, except the head should be raised enough so that the eyeball is pointing toward the ceiling. This will help keep the drops from immediately running out of the eye. The dropper should be held close to, but not touching, the eye. Drops allowed to fall onto your dog's eye from as little as one inch away can cause pain. Again, gently massage the eyelids, and keep her occupied.

As a general rule, never give your dog any medication which was intended to be taken by you. Aside from the fact that it may not work the same in dogs as in people, the obvious difference in body size and weight is almost sure to produce an overdose in your dog, which with many drugs, could be fatal. This is particularly true of tranquilizers, aspirin, pain killers, and sleeping pills. Resist the temptation to give your dog *something* to make her "more comfortable until the doctor sees her." She will probably do just as well with nothing. If you *really* think she needs something, phone your veterinarian for advice, no matter what time, or which day, it is! Too many dogs have been brought to the threshhold of death by the "temporary relief" of human medicines.

Because some of the chronic illnesses which might affect your aging dog can cause some physical discomfort, your veterinarian will occasionally prescribe *controlled* drugs, such as barbiturates or other pain killers. These will have a specially marked label printed on orange paper. Keep such medicines out of everyone's reach and, preferably, under lock and key.

In summary, here are some important Dos and Don'ts.

Do

- be sure the medication you are giving is the one prescribed for your dog and for the particular condition she now has.
- tell your present veterinarian of *any* medications prescribed by another doctor which your dog is still taking.
- follow directions meticulously.
- inform your doctor of *any* unexpected side effects.
- date all medications when you receive them if not already done.
- refrigerate medications so marked.
- transfer the label as well as the medication if you change the container it was dispensed in.
- keep all medications out of the reach of children *and your dog*.

Don't

- give medication prescribed for another dog.
- exceed the prescribed dose or frequency.
- use medication in an unlabeled container.
- remove medication from its container in a dark or dimly lit room. Many containers look and feel alike—you may give your dog the wrong drug.
- keep leftover medications unless your doctor tells you too.
- give medication previously prescribed for what "looks like the very same problem" wihout first speaking with your veterinarian.
- leave ointments near a heat source or in the sun as some may turn rancid or otherwise lose their effectiveness.

PART TWO

Specific Diseases or Disorders of the Aging Dog

This section does not purport to be a compendium of information on all disorders of the geriatric canine. Such an effort would by itself be a book of encyclopedic proportions. I have selected those conditions which are met with *primarily* in older dogs or those in which advancing age makes significant alterations in the course of the disorder. Ailments which are associated primarily with younger dogs or are unrelated to and unaffected by age have been excluded.

Please keep in mind that this section is *not* a treatise on the diagnosis and treatment of geriatric disorders, and you should *never* attempt to use it as if it were. The signs and symptoms, indicated treatments, and expected responses described herein will be applicable to most dogs who develop a particular ailment but may vary, or be quite different, if *your* dog develops that same disorder. After a thorough examination of *your* dog, your family veterinarian will diagnose what *your* dog's problem is and prescribe a course of therapy specifically for *your* dog which may be at variance with material presented here. Remember, your veterinarian can examine your dog—this book cannot!

Although there are many disorders of geriatric dogs discussed here, it does not mean that every aging dog will develop all, or even most, of them. Your dog is most likely to be affected by only a very few such disorders.

3
The Skin

The skin has ofttimes been described as an envelope which encloses and protects all the other organs of the body. Yet it does more than just that; it is itself a true organ system, and has the most direct contact with the external environment of any body organ. The skin aids in the maintenance of proper temperature and water content in your dog's body and, in addition to its own disorders, changes in its health state can reflect primary disorders in internal organs.

Dry Skin

The pliability and softness of skin is due to the water in its cells. Any prolonged significant loss of that water will produce a dry, flaky or brittle skin. The sebaceous glands in the skin, as one of their functions, form a thin emulsionlike coating over the skin's surface which helps retain the proper amount of cutaneous moisture. Diminished function of these glands commonly occurs in advancing age, as well as in illness or malnutrition, allowing surface evaporation to increase and thereby dehydrate and dry out the skin. You can help, by vigorous daily brushing, to stimulate the skin and more evenly distribute the available skin gland secretions. *Infrequent* bathing with a non-drying, non-oil removing shampoo may also help. Your family veterinarian can recommend suitable preparations available in your area.

Callouses of the Elbows and Hocks

When dogs lie down in their normal position, the major portion of their weight is supported by their elbows, especially when on hard surfaces. With the passage of sufficient time, the hair covering the elbows disappears as the constant pressure destroys the local hair follicles. In response to this same pressure the skin undergoes hyperkeratinization, a thickening and toughening process, and callouses are formed. A similar process can take place in the skin covering the hock joints, but this is less frequent. The rate at which these callouses form is directly proportional to the size and weight of your dog. They are rarely seen in Chihuahuas or other toy breeds, regardless of age, but occur with great frequency in German shepherds, Dobermans, Newfoundlands, Great Danes, and most other giant breeds as early as five years of age. As a rule they cause no problems. If they seem inordinately dry or hard, gently rubbing in a small amount of white petrolatum ointment once or twice a week should keep them soft enough to avoid any difficulties. Once in a while they do get so hard that they start to crack, developing raw fistulas which readily become infected. Your dog will lick at them and compound the problem by irritating the skin. When callouses reach this stage, they need prompt veterinary attention. One thing you can do to help prevent their occurrence, as well as aid their healing when being treated, is to provide a soft surface for your dog to lie on, thus reducing the amount of pressure.

External Parasites

Fleas, ticks, lice—these are the main parasites of the aging dog, although lice are no longer particularly common in the United States. There is no evidence to suggest that advancing years either decreases or increases susceptibility. Fleas and ticks appear to enjoy dogs of all ages. It should be remembered that fleas are the intermediate host in the life cycle of the common dog tapeworm, *Dipylidium caninum*, and that ticks can transmit a variety of bacterial, viral, rickettsial, and protozoan diseases depending on their geographic area. Engorged female ticks are also capable of making a poison which causes partial to total paralysis when it enters the blood stream.

A congenital predisposition in some dogs makes them react to the saliva of fleas when bitten by them. This results in an allergic reaction, severe itching and scratching. Following elimination of the parasites, the allergy must be treated.

The focus of concern in the mature dog is not so much the parasites, as the many insecticides available to control them, and the dog's often unexpected (idiosyncrasy) reaction to these poisons. While idiosyncrasy can occur at any age, undetected changes in the kidneys, liver, and other organs of the geriatric canine can make her a more likely candidate for such a reaction. Insecticides intended for use on dogs can be divided into four main groups:

1. naturally derived chemicals—sulfur, rotenone, pyrethrin
2. chlorinated hydrocarbons—lindane, toxaphene
3. carbamates
4. organophosphates

Each has advantages and disadvantages, but all are poisons and must be used with great care. Although you may have used just about any type in the past, when your dog is getting on in years you had best consult your veterinarian for a recommendation or prescription for one that will be both safe and effective. Follow directions explicitly! Don't forget that the premises must also be treated to get rid of the parasites. It is possible that the same preparation you use on your dog may be satisfactory for the premises, or you may need something else. Once again, ask your veterinarian.

I have here purposely avoided recommending sprays, powders, dips, collars, medallions, and so on. You or your doctor will have a preference. As long as it is safe and effective, the choice is rarely of consequence.

Wounds, Cuts, and Abrasions

When a young, healthy dog superficially cuts or otherwise injures his skin, it is not uncommon among dog owners to expect that nature will heal it successfully. This is usually what does happen, with little or no infection or scarring. In the older dog this may no longer occur. Even minor breaks in the surface of aging skin can become serious.

The lowered resistance to infection found in aging dogs exists in their skin as well as in the rest of their body systems. Movement of white blood cells to the injured site can be slowed due to problems of circulation in the surrounding blood vessels, reduced efficiency of the heart's pumping action, or insufficient numbers of white cells being produced in the aging body.

"Minor" cuts or abrasions should have the hair around them trimmed close to the skin, then be washed with plenty of mild soap and warm water. If there is any significant bleeding after the washing, it can be controlled by placing a *clean* handkerchief or sterile gauze pad on the wound and applying direct pressure to it with your hand for five minutes. This will stop virtually all minor bleeding. Apply a simple dressing—a plastic strip bandage or tape over a gauze pad—for a few days, but watch for any swelling, redness, or oozing—possible signs of infection.

In the event that the wound is more than one-half inch in length, goes through the full thickness of the skin, is a puncture, becomes infected, or continues to bleed in spite of direct pressure, have your dog seen by your veterinarian. The wound may require surgical cleaning, suturing of blood vessels, insertion of drains, or suturing of the skin.

Ear Disorders

You may be wondering why ear problems are placed under a discussion of the skin. If you stop to think about it, you will realize that the tissue which lines the ear canal is nothing more nor less than a turning in of skin into the canal. It contains the same types of cells as body skin as well as sebaceous glands and hair follicles. It is important to keep this in mind, as anything which alters the overall health of the skin can affect the health of the ears. If your dog has been prone to ear disorders, you already know that the highest incidence is in cocker spaniels, poodles, and other breeds which have either flop ears or large amounts of hair growing in the ear canal. Should you own a German shepherd, you also know that this breed is the exception, being very susceptible to ear infections without either of these predisposing circumstances.

Ears should be wiped out *daily* with dry cotton on the end of your finger or, very carefully, with a cotton-tipped applicator stick barely damp with a drop of mineral oil. I prefer the former method, but be sure your finger nail is trimmed and well covered. You will be able to clean just as well and are less likely to injure the ear canal than with an applicator stick.

The canine ear normally secretes small amounts of soft wax (cerumen) which then dries and is slowly moved to the upper part of the ear canal by your dog's normal occasional head shaking. With daily cleaning, you will be able to remove most of that wax thus preventing ninety percent of ear problems. More important, if a problem should arise, you will know about it right away and be able to obtain professional attention before it becomes a serious or chronic one.

Hair growing in the ear canal acts as a mechanical barrier to the movement and drying of normal wax. The wax becomes trapped in the hair which then becomes matted. This effectively prevents air from circulating through the canal, the wax remains moist, the matted hair annoys the dog, and she starts scratching the ears and excessively shaking the head. This trauma irritates the ear canal lining, and it responds by producing more wax. The cycle rapidly becomes self-perpetuating. Because the environment of the canal is now very moist, even soupy, and quite warm, it is very conducive to the growth of bacteria, and an ear infection is the result. For these reasons I believe ear hair should be removed every day along with wiping out the canal. This should be done as part of the daily grooming procedure. Only a few hairs should be removed each day, and you should use only your fingers, not a tweezer or forceps. The hairs must be snapped out, as one would pluck an eyebrow, not tugged or pulled at. Properly done, there is virtually no real discomfort, and you will not cause any ear irritation.

The treatment of ear infections will vary greatly from one case to another because of the wide spectrum of bacteria and fungi that can be involved. There exists a plethora of medications intended for the treatment of ear disorders, perhaps more than for any other canine ailment. Each is effective in its own way in selected cases. Treatment is essentially the same in aging dogs as in younger ones and will not be dealt with here. Nevertheless, the ear canal of older dogs, like their skin, is less resistant to infection and may take longer to respond to therapy, requiring a little more of your time and patience.

Allergies

Some years ago it seemed fashionable to have "an allergy," but there was precious little ego satisfaction to be garnered from the discomfort it caused. Individually, dogs probably do not suffer from as many allergic reactions as people, but they certainly do have allergies. The establishment in this country of the Academy of Veterinary Allergy almost a decade ago surely attests to that fact. Although the knowledge of veterinary allergy has grown by leaps and bounds during this time, the accurate diagnosis of the cause, and the successful treatment, of allergic conditions still leaves something to be desired.

We are all familiar with the common symptoms of many allergies—itchy skin, hives, runny itchy eyes, sneezing, diarrhea—and with a good history from you, your veterinarian will be able to diagnose when the problem is indeed an allergy. But trying to find the *specific* cause of an allergic reaction can often be like hunting for the proverbial needle in a haystack! Literally anything your dog is exposed to could become an antigen or allergen—substances which when introduced into your dog's body sensitize him by stimulating the production of antibodies. Some dogs are more predisposed to this process than others and can be sensitized by a single exposure, while others require numerous contacts with the same antigen before sensitization develops. A few lucky ones may never become sensitized. Once sensitized, however, subsequent exposure causes a reaction between the antigen and the antibody developed against it, and an allergic reaction is produced. This may happen immediately or can be delayed for several hours or days.

Predisposed dog + allergen ⟶ antibodies + subsequent allergen ⟶ allergic reaction
Normal dog + allergen ⟶ no antibodies + subsequent allergen ⟶ no allergic reaction

There are basically two ways of trying to find the specific cause of an allergy—elimination trials, a sort of trial-and-error method, and specific allergen skin testing, a somewhat more scientific trial-and-error method. Both are time consuming, require a great deal of patience and diligent following of instructions, and may fail to yield complete answers. In addition, skin testing can be expensive.

Should it be suspected that the allergen is in the food, the diet will be changed immediately to a one-food type. Since most dogs are not fed lamb regularly, this meat will often serve as the basic test diet since your dog would not likely be allergic to it. If the allergy symptoms disappear, you can be fairly sure the problem is in the diet. Taking one food element at a time from your dog's regular diet, it is added to the lamb and fed for five to seven days. No reaction? That food is OK. If there is a reaction which disappears when that food item is again eliminated, you have discovered something your dog is allergic to. It may not be the only food allergen, however, so all elements of the customary diet should be tested.

The detective problem is infinitely more difficult when the allergen is believed to be in the environment. This includes inhaled as well as direct physical contact substances. It is not easy to eliminate single items from a dog's environment and, in difficult cases, your veterinarian may advise hospitalization for several days. This would certainly be quite an environmental change, and many times the allergy disappears with no further diagnostics or treatments. In other cases it turns into a by-guess-and-by-gosh search at home. Is it that wool blanket Gypsy sleeps on or the highly polished wax floor, carefully done every week, on which she takes her afternoon nap? Is it the fumes from your basement furnace or the pollen in your backyard, or could it be the chemical dye in the sweater or blanket you've put on her for the winter? It goes on and on, and in many cases the answer is stumbled upon only by accident.

Eventually it may be necessary to have Gypsy skin-tested for the common, and not so common, canine allergens. Unless your family veterinarian is trained in this comparatively new technique, she will probably refer you and Gypsy to a colleague who is a trained dermatologist or allergist. It may require leaving Gypsy for a few days or returning with her a number of times. Patience and understanding of the doctor's very difficult diagnostic problem is an important asset for you.

During all the elimination trials or skin testing, the doctor will, of course, try to relieve the symptoms of the allergy and make Gypsy more comfortable. There may be injections or oral medication of antihistamines or corticosteroids, depending on whether it is an immediate or delayed allergy; lotions or ointments to be used on the skin; and perhaps some eye medication. One of the most difficult of all the problems in sleuthing out the causative agent is that symptomatic treatment must be stopped during the test period. This means Gypsy will have to be taken off all medication at least forty-eight hours or more before the testing starts. If symptoms recur severely enough, the testing may have to be stopped temporarily while medication is given again. Once the cause is determined, it should be permanently eliminated and therapy continued until Gypsy is completely normal. This could take several weeks!

In human medicine it has been possible to desensitize some allergic people by giving them a series of injections before they are exposed. Hay fever allergy is an example most of us are familiar with. This procedure has had fairly good results in dogs also, with nearly three-fourths of the desensitized patients obtaining complete or almost complete relief from their allergies. However, it is sometimes necessary to repeat the injections for two or three years in a row to get permanent relief. An occasional dog will require desensitization every year for the remainder of its life. As with skin testing, you will probably be referred to a veterinary allergist or dermatologist for desensitization. Short of this procedure, we must depend on preventing further contact with a known allergen in order to avoid the unwelcome symptoms of allergies.

Seborrhea

Despite tremendous advances in dermatology over the last two decades, seborrhea continues to be one of the most puzzling and frustrating disorders of the skin. It is a chronic, often lifelong, disease which can be alleviated and improved, but which cannot be cured with our present knowledge. It occurs in both a dry form; common in Irish setters, dachshunds and German shepherds, and an oily form; most frequently seen in cocker and springer spaniels, especially the blonde cocker spaniels. Dogs with the dry form develop grayish-white dry scales—dandruff—which are not at all oily and are distributed throughout the haircoat. The oily form is far more distressing to both dog and owner. The skin exhibits greasy, scaly deposits which stick to and mat the hair. A characteristic rancid fat odor is one of the unpleasant signs of this form of the disease. At its worst, the oily form is accompanied by severe itching and reddening of the skin.

This disagreeable condition is a frequent secondary complication in many skin and nonskin disorders such as fungal infections, severe flea or tick infestation, dermal allergies, insufficient dietary fat or deficient utilization of it, as well as in low thyroid gland output. It can also be a complication in the female hormonal abnormality known as ovarian imbalance and in the male hypoandrogenism or feminizing syndrome. In each of these, the primary disorder must be corrected before any treatment of the seborrhea can be undertaken.

These dogs with true primary seborrhea have no known cause for it. At least we are unable to determine any cause. Therapy is directed at getting rid of the crusts and dandruff, reducing the greasiness and rancid odor, and alleviating the itching and scratching. Fat supplementation is indicated but must be carefully evaluated in light of your dog's ability to properly digest fats. Special shampoos containing sulfur, salicylic acid, or coal tar derivatives will be prescribed and should be applied once weekly in most cases. They are used in the same manner as outlined earlier under Grooming, but with one important exception. When completely lathered and rubbed in thoroughly, the antiseborrheic shampoo must be allowed to remain in contact with the dog's skin for ten to fifteen minutes by the clock, before rinsing it off. For those dogs with the dry form of this disease, the shampoo should be followed by an emollient bath oil such as Alpha-Keri® or a similar product. A mixture of two capfuls in one-half gallon of warm water is *gently* rubbed in all over the dog and allowed to remain without rinsing. Drying should be thorough but very gentle.

Dogs who have the additional problems of itchiness and redness may be given cortisone-like medication to provide relief. The dose will be kept as low as will control the annoying symptoms and frequently can be discontinued for brief periods. This will help avoid occasional side effects of prolonged treatment with these drugs, such as increased thirst, appetite, and urination.

You should understand that although seborrhea cannot be cured, the problems it causes you and your dog can almost always be controlled satisfactorily by conscientious adherence to the prescribed routine of shampoos, diet supplementation, and grooming. You must not expect too much, too soon, or you will quickly become frustrated and disappointed. Great patience, love, and commitment are necessary to bring about a reasonable compromise between your dog's health needs and your life patterns. For an example of what I mean, read about Hank in the first of Three Love Stories in the appendix.

Anal Sacs

These paired structures, sometimes referred to as anal glands, are invaginations of the skin located on either side of, and slightly below, the anus. Each has a narrow duct which opens onto the inner edge of the anus. These sacs are found in many four-legged animals but in the dog have no function of which we are aware. Unfortunately, they do produce an unpleasant pungent-smelling fluid secretion which is emptied periodically during the act of defecation. In the older dog, the secretion can become viscous or pasty, making it increasingly difficult for the sacs to be emptied. The area over the affected sac or sacs becomes swollen and painful, and the skin becomes reddened. As the pressure of the thickening secretion increases, the dog becomes aware of it and will either scoot its rear along the ground or chew somewhere in its hind quarters, trying to relieve the pressure. Inasmuch as few dogs can actually reach their anus, they will chew on the stifle, flank, groin, tail, hind feet—wherever they think chewing will relieve the sensations they are experiencing.

Your veterinarian should be visited at this point, so he can properly empty the sacs and relieve the itchiness. If the problem is a recurrent one, as is seen in a few dogs, he may be able to teach you how correctly and safely to do this messy job at home. It is very difficult to explain in writing, and I shall not attempt to. Allowing the sacs to continue to fill and go untreated will result in your dog creating a severe secondary dermatitis from the biting and scratching of the skin.

Neglected abnormal anal sacs eventually become abscessed, necessitating surgical drainage and sometimes hospitalization. In some cases the gentle application of hot moist compresses to the swollen but unbroken abscess for several days might soften the viscous contents and open the duct enough to permit drainage through its natural opening. If you're lucky and it works, you can avoid an operation. In the event it cannot drain out through the duct, the abscess may break open through the skin and the pus or blood-tinged contents will ooze out. This does *not* solve the problem; the broken abscess should have professional follow-up which may include surgical cleaning, packing, or antibiotics.

Once in a while, a dog will develop a chronic problem with its anal sacs, and your veterinarian may advise surgically removing the sacs. A few days of hospital care may be needed, but there is relatively little aftercare on your part nor will the operation affect your dog's behavior.

Tumors

It is not known why there is a greater incidence of skin tumors in mature and aging dogs, but such growths account for almost thirty-five percent of all tumors reported in canines. Over a period of many years, exposure of the skin to the ultraviolet rays of the sun, various chemical pollutants, or other carcinogens (cancer producing substances) may have some relationship, but this is not as yet well documented. We do know that the incidence is significantly higher in certain breeds—Boston, wirehaired and Scottish terriers, cocker spaniels, and boxers—but here too, the specific reasons are unknown.

Sebaceous gland adenoma is probably the commonest skin tumor of older dogs. They can occur anywhere on the body but seem to have a preference for the legs, head, and neck. These tumors are firm to the touch, grey to pink in color, and have a lobulated, cauliflower-like elevated appearance. This type of adenoma is *benign* and generally of no consequence. They can be unsightly and possibly annoy your dog, depending on their location. Should he scratch at them he can traumatize the tumors, introduce infection, and perhaps stimulate abnormal growth. If your dog is not bothered by them and doesn't scratch or lick them, they can be left alone. Care, however, must be taken to avoid them when brushing your dog. In the event he is bothering such adenomas, they start growing rapidly, or there are many of them over his body, making grooming difficult, they can be removed surgically with great success. There is virtually no aftercare.

Sammy, an eleven-year-old poodle, had such an adenoma, about an inch in diameter, near the base of his tail for three months and wouldn't leave it alone. A veterinarian in another part of the country who had examined it orginally was reluctant to operate "due to the dog's advanced age," even though Sammy was damaging the tumor and the skin around it. Upon his return to New York, the adenoma was removed under a safe, short-acting anesthetic, and he went home the same day. Except for removal of the stitches a week later, there was no aftercare. The sebaceous gland adenoma on the eyelid of another eleven-year-old poodle, named Dizzy, did require a few days hospital care, mainly to keep him from scratching at, and removing, the stitches and the protective bandage.

A similar-appearing tumor, the *papilloma,* or wart, is also quite commonly seen. It is generally one centimeter or less in size with a thickened, somewhat crusty surface, and is found with much greater frequency in males than in females. Everything else mentioned above about the sebaceous gland adenoma, often incorrectly called "warts," is equally true of papillomas.

The *perianal gland tumor* is a more serious and unsightly growth. There are specialized sebaceous cells in these glands which surround the anus of the dog. Like anal sacs, they have no known function but often produce nodular growths which become inflamed, ulcerated, infected, and develop fistulas. Because of occasional physical discomfort and for mechanical reasons, these tumors frequently interfere to some degree with defecation. This causes additional soiling of the perianal tissue and increases the difficulty of keeping the area clean. Gentle washing with warm water after each bowel movement, before bedtime, and first thing in the morning will help keep the odors to a minimum and the tissues acceptably clean. This tumor occurs almost exclusively in males and most often in fox terriers and cocker spaniels. They are rarely malignant and virtually never metastasize (spread to other parts of the body).

Complete early surgical removal is the best treatment and is almost always successful. In advanced, or neglected, cases in which tumors completely encircle the anus, a so-called "donut" operation may be required. It is a more complicated procedure but yields equally good results, although a rare case may lose some control of its bowels. Because these tumors are hormone related, it is important that the dog be castrated to prevent recurrence and growth of new tumors. The use of female hormones in place of castration gives only temporary results and requires prolonged repeated use which, with estrogens, can have undesirable side effects. As soon as the estrogens are stopped, the tumor regrows. In the rare advanced case, which is so longer operable, radiation therapy is very effective as perianal gland tumors are quite radiosensitive.

Pepe, a thirteen-year-old wirehair fox terrier with chronic kidney disease of four years duration, had a three-year-old perianal gland tumor. I had been unable to convince the owner to let me operate when the tumor was first diagnosed and quite small. She was certain that a dog of ten "couldn't live through it." When she could no longer cope with the mess and foul odors from the tumor, she gave in. Pepe had a "donut" operation and was castrated, returning home in just four days. Bowel control remained normal, and his failing kidneys held out for almost three years more.

There are several other types of skin tumors which are more dangerous, but all of them are most benefited by early surgical removal. I have divided the more common ones into three groups based on prognosis.

Good surgical prognosis:

Basal cell carcinoma—usually a single, hard tumor, ¼–1 inch in size, with a higher incidence in cocker spaniels. Radiosensitive. Rarely metastasize.

Mastocytoma—a round, hairless swelling, not movable within the skin. Can occur anywhere on the body. Common in Boston terriers and boxers. Radiosensitive. Little metastasis if removed early. Later metastasize very readily.

Neurofibroma—usually a cluster of small tumors under the skin of the abdomen and chest. Rarely metastasize, but sometimes recur after surgery. Once in a while these tumors disappear by themselves.

Poor surgical prognosis:

Squamous cell carcinoma—a thickened round skin growth anywhere on the body, but frequently on the lips, toes, scrotum and torso. Ulcerates rapidly. Readily metastasizes.

Fibrosarcoma—small tumors about the head, breasts and legs which grow rapidly and ulcerate. Highly malignant, they metastasize readily, especially to the lungs.

Rapidly terminal in most cases:

Melanoma—a tumor of the pigment cells in the skin. A round, black and smooth growth, especially on the mouth, feet, and eyelids. Often has a velvety feel. Seen frequently in Scottish and Boston terriers. Rapid metastasis. Many are resistant to radiation therapy.

Cutaneous lymphosarcoma—can be primary in the skin or secondary to lymphosarcoma elsewhere in the body. See pages 205–206 for a full discussion of canine lymphosarcoma.

These last two highly malignant tumors rarely permit a survival time of more than three to six months and are generally unresponsive to any kind of treatment. Palliative therapy to keep the dog comfortable is reasonably effective until the very end. Wet applications or soaking baths, if advised by your veterinarian, can also be very comforting to a dog with cutaneous lymphosarcoma.

4
The Digestive System

It has been said that some eat to live while others live to eat. Be that as it may, eating and drinking are essential to life, and it is the job of the digestive system to convert food and water from their ingested form into forms that can be absorbed into the body to provide essential nutrients. It also must eliminate waste products and resorb fluid from them.

The digestive system is little more than a hollow tube with several outpouchings; it extends from one end of the body to the other and has several functionally associated other organs. Starting with the mouth and including the teeth, tongue, and salivary glands, the system continues with the esophagus, stomach, small intestine, cecum, colon or large intestine, and the rectum, ending at the anus. Some of the functions of the pancreas, liver, and gall bladder are intimately involved in the absorption of food and water and, to that extent, these organs are considered part of the digestive system.

Dentistry

Dental problems are one of the commonest ailments of the older dog. In spite of this, you can make a major contribution to your dog's general health by practicing preventive dental care at home. When your dog reached six or seven months of age, he had forty-two adult teeth consisting of three incisors, one canine, four premolars, and two molars on each side of the upper jaw. The lower jaw was the same, except that there were three molars on each side. In many of the short-faced breeds like the pug, Boston terrier, and English bulldog, the last molars may be missing. Depending upon your past diligence, all or few of those original adult teeth may now remain in your dog's mouth.

Adult Dental Formula

	Right Side	Left Side
Upper Jaw	M M P P P P C I I I	I I I C P P P P M M
Lower Jaw	M M M P P P P C I I I	I I I C P P P P M M M

Dogs tend to tear their food with the four long canine teeth (fangs) and swallow it. Unlike cats and people, they rarely chew food unless a piece is very large or is too tough to tear. In the wild, most natural foods were in this latter category and required lots of chewing. The foods fed dogs today are usually gulped down. As a result, your dog is far more likely to have dental problems, unless you do something to help him.

There are many types of bacteria normally living in a dog's mouth, but they are kept under control by the protective action of the gingival epithelium—the gum-lining membrane—and its immune defense mechanism. A breakdown in this mechanism, improper diet, inadequate chewing, food particle accumulation, mechanical injury to the gums, or an inadequate oral hygiene program can allow these previously harmless bacteria to multiply out of control. Periodontal disease or pyorrhea, the most common infectious process in the oral cavity, is the result.

In the early stage of periodontal disease, only slight redness of the gumline may be visible. If you are following the dental hygiene program described below, this is the stage at which you will be able to detect the problem and have it treated before it gets worse. In the later stages, gum recession, halitosis, tartar, or dental calculus deposits which may completely cover a tooth, pus along the gums or between the teeth, exposed roots, and loose teeth become all too readily apparent. The toxins produced by the bacteria at this stage can be absorbed into the body and affect other organs, such as the liver and kidneys.

Good dental care starts at home with you. Your dog should be fed a diet which encourages her to do more than just gulp down the food. Dry foods, not the semimoist kind, in either kibble, nugget, biscuit, or "bone" form should be fed daily along with any meat foods. Rawhide chew toys, now available in a seemingly endless variety of sizes and shapes, are an absolute must. It is a rare dog who will not play with, and endlessly chew on, such a toy. This provides a massaging action to the gums and helps loosen food particles from between the teeth. In addition, because it is made of animal tissue, the rawhide will digest when she swallows pieces of it, thereby making it a safe as well as a useful toy.

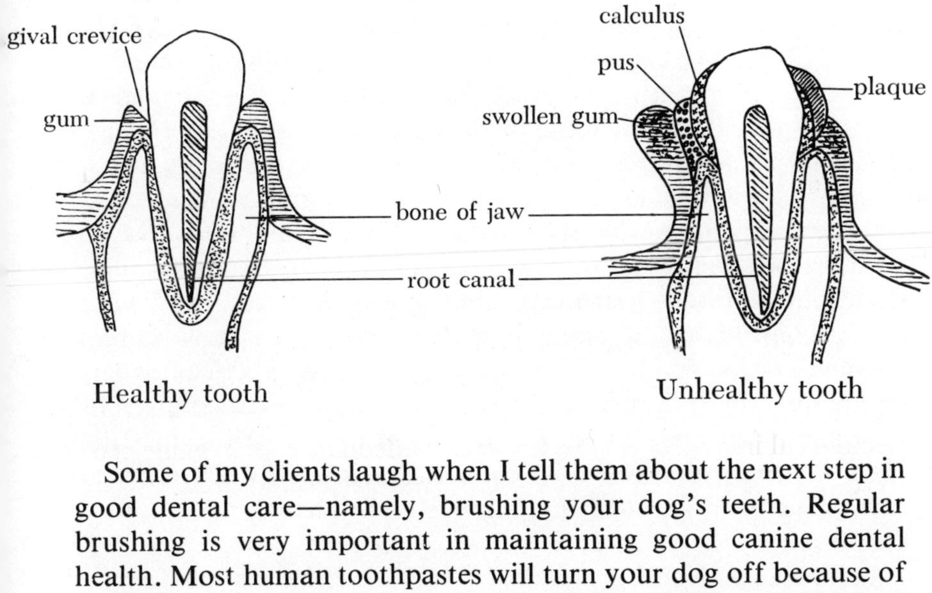

Healthy tooth

Unhealthy tooth

Some of my clients laugh when I tell them about the next step in good dental care—namely, brushing your dog's teeth. Regular brushing is very important in maintaining good canine dental health. Most human toothpastes will turn your dog off because of the flavorings and detergents they contain, and the majority of dental powders are too abrasive. The dentifrice of choice is baking soda (sodium bicarbonate). Your bare finger, with fingernail carefully trimmed and cleaned, is used to apply the powder. I do not recommend a toothbrush, or even a cloth over your finger, as you are more likely to accidentally injure the gums, cheek, and tongue with them than with your bare finger. Simply moisten your finger, dip it in the dry baking soda, and start brushing. At first, do only two or three teeth at a time, gradually increasing the number each day. Most dogs will eventually let you do the entire mouth at one time.

The brushing should be done about one hour after feeding and, in the geriatric dog, every day. It will take practice and patience to succeed. The outside of the teeth will be easy to reach, but the inner surfaces will present more of a problem, requiring opening of the mouth and placing your finger and hand inside it. Your dog's tongue will continually try to push your finger away from its goal. But work at it! Calculus and plaque accumulate on the inner, as well as the outer, surfaces of the teeth.

Many dogs who, like people, are prone to tartar deposits, will, due to individual metabolic and hereditary variations, develop periodontal desease even with good home care. This is the time to have your family veterinarian do a complete dental prophylaxis, which will remove calculus and plaque, clean the gingival crevice, and scale and smooth the surfaces of the teeth and the subgingival areas. If a tooth is very loose or the gum over it so badly receded that the root is exposed and infected, it may be necessary to extract it. In a neglected mouth, it is not uncommon to have to extract several teeth during a prophylaxis. If they cannot be salvaged as described below in the final paragraph on Dentistry, they should be removed. Left in the mouth, they will only cause your dog discomfort at best, and pain at worst, as well as provide areas for bacteria and food particles again to accumulate. Do not worry about your dog's ability to eat even after many extractions. The very habit that contributed to the loss of those teeth in the first place—namely, that few dogs chew their food—will allow her to eat satisfactorily, even if the only teeth she has left are the four canines!

Following a dental prophylaxis, your veterinarian may advise you to feed a soft diet for a few days to a week. Use your dog's regular diet, but put it in a blender with a bit of water and make an oatmeal-like paste of it. You should also wash the mouth after each meal using a mild salt solution applied with a small *soft* cloth. Dab it on—do not rub the gums. They will be quite tender for several days and may bleed slightly after eating or even drinking. There is no need to worry about this unless the bleeding becomes excessive. Obviously her teeth should not be brushed until the gums have healed. In the event the gums were badly infected, your veterinarian may also prescribe an antibiotic for several days. Be sure to give it for the full time prescribed.

It is good preventive medicine for your geriatric dog to have a complete dental prophylaxis once a year. Some individuals may require it more or less frequently to maintain good health. The general anesthesia usually needed to do the prophylaxis properly should not present any undue risk, even in the aging dog, what with the greater safety of today's newer anesthetics.

Watch your dog for extra-oral signs of dental problems. Should your dog start to eat, stop suddenly and perhaps drop some of the food from his mouth, suspect a painful loose or infected tooth. If he paws at his mouth look inside for the cause. If he spends an unusual amount of time licking his lips after eating, or he works his tongue over and over his teeth, carefully examine the mouth for food particles stuck between the teeth. Look also for tartar rubbing against the gums or cheeks, swelling along the gums (which could be an abscess), red and inflamed gums, overgrown gums, and loose or infected teeth. A swelling just below his eye is very likely the result of an abscess of the root of the fourth premolar tooth, which has eroded into the sinus cavity below that eye. In any of these circumstances, you should have your dog examined as soon as possible by your veterinarian.

Dogs do not get cavities with anywhere near the frequency of people, and that is certainly fortunate. When found, however, they tend to be on or near an exposed root. If the rest of the tooth is in good health, the cavity can be treated and filled. Root canal work and other restorative procedures such as crowning, while not done by all veterinarians, is generally available in most areas from one who has a special interest in dentistry. Should you choose to have this work done on your dog, your veterinarian will refer you to a colleague, if he does not do this type of dentistry himself. Thus, broken and chipped teeth, as well as infected ones, can often be restored instead of being extracted. The majority of dogs will tolerate the new materials currently used in these procedures, which will last for many years. The pros and cons of having such work performed on your dog's mouth is beyond the scope of this book and must be based on the individual assessment of each patient.

Vomiting and Diarrhea

Although they occur with considerable frequency, vomiting and diarrhea rarely are diseases in and of themselves but rather are symptoms of disorders in either the stomach or intestines, or in other parts of the body. Fear, middle ear infection, and kidney disease can stimulate vomiting while hyperexcitability, generalized infections, congestive heart failure, and intestinal parasites may cause diarrhea. There are many other diverse contributing causes of these two gastrointestinal symptoms. By observing the color and consistency of the diarrhea or the vomitus, as well as the time relationship between vomiting and eating or drinking, you will be able to help your veterinarian start down the diagnostic trail.

A vomiting dog loses large amounts of body fluid and body salt. He will frequently attempt to immediately eat and drink again, resulting in repeated vomiting and the further loss of salt and fluid. Diarrhea causes similar fluid and salt losses, and the excess drinking will likely prolong the diarrhea. An immediate first aid measure you should take until you can get your dog to your doctor's office is to remove *all* food and water.

Constipation, Obstipation, and Flatulence

As your dog grows older, the muscles of the colon and rectum may lose some of their ability to propel and expel feces adequately during a bowel movement. Reduction in stomach and intestinal digestive secretions can produce a bulkier, firmer stool as can diets very high in dry food content if there is insufficient water intake. Your dog will squat and strain to force the fecal mass slowly out. She may cry from the discomfort, there may be fresh blood on the stool or around the anus, or the stool may just protrude from but not pass out of the anus. In the latter case applying Vaseline or K–Y lubricating jelly around the anus as you gently pull on the fecal mass will usually enable you to remove it with relatively little pain to your dog.

Prostatic disease can mechanically cause constipation as the prostate gland enlarges and presses up against the floor of the rectum. Similarly, tumors in the rectum or on the anus can interfere with the passage of feces.

Any dog may have an isolated difficult bowel movement on occasion. This should be no cause for alarm if he is otherwise in good health and there is no bleeding or excessive pain. Frequent signs of constipation, however, should hie you to your family veterinarian to determine the cause and, if possible, have it corrected. Repeated bouts of constipation can slowly stretch the rectal muscles, causing permanent dilatation and resulting in chronic constipation (obstipation). Once this occurs, your dog will need frequent enemas as well as fecal softeners to help him eliminate. The increased time the stool remains in the colon and rectum will allow bacteria that normally live there to act on the stool, causing putrefaction and excessive gas production. The disagreeable flatulence (gas) will make you acutely aware of the problem. Reducing the amount of meat in his diet and exercising him more, commensurate with his health status, may help decrease the amount of flatulence.

Tumors

Advancing years may bring with them tumors of the mouth, stomach, or intestines which occur most often between ages nine and sixteen. Oral tumors are quite common, can be found on the lips, gums, or tongue, and are usually pigmented or nonpigmented malignant melanomas. It is important that any change you observe in the shape, size, or color of your dog's oral tissues be quickly brought to the attention of your veterinarian, as some tumors of the mouth can be successfully removed if done early. Prolonged growth will allow the malignant tumor to spread to nearby lymph nodes or other organs, to ulcerate and become infected, or erode into the jawbone, all of which can effectively preclude surgical removal. Early signs might include inappropriate salivation, hesitancy or difficulty in eating, and an unpleasant odor to the mouth. Since tooth and gum disorders can cause similar-appearing symptoms, the mouth should be thoroughly examined to determine the true cause.

When Cindy was presented for examination, the half-inch tumor on her lower lip had been noticed for just one week. A friendly ten-year-old part cocker spaniel, she was otherwise in good health except for repeated false pregnancies. The tumor and considerable healthy lip around it were removed, producing a slight distortion of the lip when it healed. Biopsies were taken of the nearest lymph nodes and submitted, along with the tumor, to a pathologist. Happily, both biopsies were negative, because the pathologist reported the tumor to be a malignant melanoma. No further treatment was needed and, three years later, there was still no sign of recurrence or new tumor development elsewhere.

Tumors of the stomach and intestines are less successfully treated, as they usually become quite extensive before persistent vomiting, loss of appetite, diarrhea, weight loss, or other symptoms develop. On rare occasions it may be possible to remove sections of the stomach or intestines if X-ray studies show the tumor to be small or isolated. For the others, chemotherapy may help alleviate the symptoms temporarily. There is little else that can be done except to keep such dogs comfortable for the short while that is possible.

Intestinal Parasites

"Doctor," you may ask, "only puppies and young dogs have worms, so why are you discussing it here?" This is largely true, as adult dogs tend to develop a resistance to most intestinal parasites. That doesn't mean they don't have worms, however, but only that they have comparatively few, and the worms do not thrive too well. Any stress which lowers that resistance can result in a case of worms as bad as, or worse than, is found in puppies. In the aged dog, almost any illness or debility is enough to do this. In view of this, it would seem wise to have your dog's stool checked microscopically at least once a year.

The most common intestinal parasites found in the United States are roundworms, hookworms, tapeworms, whipworms, and coccidia. All of these parasites, except tapeworms, are picked up by ingestion of infected feces either directly or indirectly. Your dog can step in a contaminated stool from another dog and later clean her feet by licking them, thus swallowing the parasite eggs. Tapeworms are transmitted through a variety of intermediate host animals in which their larvae develop. One such intermediate host is the common flea.

There are few, if any, symptoms which can specifically diagnose the presence of intestinal worms in your dog. That is why your veterinarian should examine your dog's feces microscopically to detect the presence of parasite eggs. Sometimes roundworms are either vomited or passed out with a bowel movement—they resemble varying lengths of spaghetti—but even though this makes the diagnosis, it is important to know how heavy is the infestation, so a fecal analysis should still be done. Tapeworms are segmented like a chain of beads, and sometimes individual segments will break off and crawl out of the rectum onto the surface of the anus, where they die after a short time. Your dog may try to lick them or rub them off. Whipworms live primarily in the cecum, a blind end pouch located where the small and large intestines join. They can cause severe irritation of the cecum and intermittent colitis. Whipworm-infected dogs frequently lick or bite at their right flank. Hookworms and coccidia can cause abdominal cramps, vomiting, diarrhea, constipation, coughing, blood in the stool, anemia, or no visible symptoms despite the damage they are doing internally.

With the advent of the many newer and safer worm medications now available, even geriatric dogs can be effectively freed from intestinal parasites.

Liver Disease

Physically the largest organ in the body other than the intestines, the liver is also the busiest, being involved in literally *hundreds* of widely differing metabolic functions necessary for the sustaining of life. These include the building of body proteins; processing and storing carbohydrates; rendering harmless many drugs, chemicals, and poisons; metabolizing fats; and the formation of bile needed for the proper digestion of foods, to name just a very few. Because the liver is so vital to survival and yet is constantly at work, nature has seen fit to give it a tremendous ability to regenerate new tissue when damaged during any of its multitudinous functions. Unlike the kidneys, brain, and many other organs of the body, the liver can be injured, damaged, and poisoned—often repeatedly—and still its huge reserve capacity enables it, more or less, to maintain the body's normal status quo.

Specific symptoms of early liver disease are therefore, of necessity, vague or nonexistent. As much as sixty to seventy percent of that organ can be severely damaged before clear-cut evidence becomes apparent. Symptoms such as vomiting, diarrhea, loss of appetite, anemia, lethargy, abdominal fluid, and even jaundice can all be found in disorders of other organs and body systems, as well as in liver disease. To complicate matters further, there can be symptoms which seem clearly to point elsewhere, such as bone abnormalities, neurologic disease, hormone imbalances, and blood disorders, which in reality are the result of liver disease.

Because of these problems, your veterinarian will often not be able readily or definitively to diagnose the liver as the source of your dog's illness. There are, however, two physical findings which, if present, will direct his interest toward that organ. If he can feel that your dog's liver is enlarged or swollen, or he finds the feces to be extremely light or gray in color, his attention will zero in on the liver and blood tests, X rays, and other diagnostic procedures to help confirm the diagnosis.

Disorders of the liver can be produced by viral or bacterial infections, poisons such as arsenic, mercury, copper, carbon tetrachloride, the phosphorus in old-fashioned wooden matches, or by tumors. Cirrhosis, a scarring and destruction of liver tissue, the source of which is poorly understood, is another cause of liver malfunction. Because of this organ's hundreds of activities, there can be almost as many factors contributing to the production of liver disease; the symptoms and treatments varying with each factor. For these reasons, I leave a full discussion of the symptoms, problems, and therapy of liver disease to your family veterinarian.

5
The Reproductive System

There are relatively few serious disorders of the canine reproductive system peculiar to or seen with increased frequency in the aging dog. But these disorders are rather common occurrences in many older dogs and are potentially life threatening. In the female dog two such conditions, mammary gland tumors and pyometra, as well as the less serious false pregnancy and mismating, can be prevented to varying degrees, as discussed further on, by ovariohysterectomy. If your dog has already had such surgery you have removed the sources of several major threats to her continuing good health. Although castration of the male will similarly prevent at least two reproductive disorders related to aging, side effects are more extensive and such surgery is rarely recommended for preventive reasons. The treatment of existing reproductive disease may, however, require such an operation.

Balanoposthitis

This inflammation of the penis and prepuce (sheath) is seen with variable frequency in dogs of all ages, even young puppies, but is observed increasingly in aging males. Small amounts of yellow or grayish discharge at the opening of the prepuce are apparent although the dog's licking at the area may clean most of it away. In severer cases, the amount of discharge is quite large and will be greenish and puslike, often matting the surrounding abdominal hair in long-coated dogs. The surface of the penis and the lining of the prepuce develop multiple little bumps, called lymphoid follicles, and bacteria actively begin to grow in the secretions. Should your dog have this problem, you will often find some of the discharge on the various surfaces that he lies on for any length of time.

You can usually clear up mild cases yourself by gently flushing out the sheath twice daily with hydrogen peroxide solution for a week or ten days. Using a rubber human ear syringe to hold the peroxide, insert its tip into the sheath opening, at the same time pulling the sheath gently toward the syringe. This will avoid the syringe tip touching the penis. Holding the sheath opening firmly around the syringe tip, slowly instill the peroxide until the prepuce distends *slightly*. Remove the syringe, keeping the prepuce opening closed, and gently massage the fluid back and forth within the sheath. Release the opening, let the fluid drain out, and carefully clean the surrounding area.

More severe cases should be treated by your veterinarian and may require the application of irritating medications to these delicate tissues. This would, of course, be done under anesthesia and probably followed with soothing antibiotic ointments which you would continue at home as instructed.

Your older dog may be recurrently bothered by balanoposthitis. Regular flushing with peroxide or the application of an antibiotic ointment or both, done once or twice weekly should keep the discharge under control and avoid the more serious problems.

Disorders of the Prostate Gland

Hyperplasia of the prostate gland is a benign enlargement due to an increase in the number of cells within the gland and occurs in about two-thirds of older male dogs. However, only a small percentage of these dogs ever show any noticeable signs of the abnormality. The underlying cause is unknown but is thought to be an imbalance of the hormones produced in aging testicles. As the prostate is located directly below the rectum, the enlarged gland may press up against the rectal wall and cause difficulty and discomfort while defecating, straining, and constipation. Unlike man, there is rarely any pain or difficulty in urinating.

Medical treatment with an estrogen injection generally stops the symptoms, reduces the size of the prostate within five or six days, and will keep it that way for several months, in most cases, and occasionally for several years. Some few dogs respond poorly, or not at all, and can be helped only by castration, which causes a permanent shrinking of the prostate. Should your dog need this operation, he will be home from the hospital in just a few days, but you should keep him quiet and resting for at least one week. A low-bulk diet may be advised for several days. He will probably walk cautiously at first, experiencing some slight discomfort each time he moves a rear leg. This may prompt him to lick or bite at the stitches. Restraint collars or tranquilizers may be used for a short time until the operation is healed and the stitches can be removed.

Cancer of the prostate is rare in dogs and fortunately so. By the time any noticeable symptoms develop, the tumor has almost always spread to other parts of the body, making it inoperable. Severe loss of weight, lameness in one or both rear legs, pain and difficulty during urination, blood at the beginning of urination, and low back pain may be present in addition to difficult defecation and constipation. Castration or estrogen therapy offer temporary relief of symptoms, but the tumor continues on its destructive course. A recent discovery holds out hope that immunotherapy may be successfully used to treat prostatic cancer but such research is still in its infancy.

Tumors of the Testicles

More than three-fourths of all testicular tumors are found in older dogs and can involve one or both testicles. Though tumors can develop from any of the three distinct types of cells found in the normal canine testicle, each produces rather firm nodular enlargements which may be as little as one-fourth inch to as much as four inches in diameter. The larger ones will make it difficult or painful for the dog to walk. While not every swelling or enlargement of the scrotum or testicles is a tumor, *all* such increases in size are potentially serious and should be brought to the attention of your veterinarian as quickly as possible.

In the early stages, a slight enlargement may be the only external sign. With time, however, very obvious and disconcerting symptoms can occur. Poor hair growth, hair that is brittle, and a symmetrical loss of hair from the underside of the chest and abdomen and the backs and sides of the thighs develop. The hairless skin gets thin and soft to the touch. The nipples of the breasts get larger and may even produce a thin watery fluid. This group of symptoms is frequently referred to as the "male feminization syndrome" and the dog can actually become attractive to other male dogs.

Other signs seen with testicular tumors include a slight swelling of the prepuce, giving it a tendency to sag or hang rather loosely. The penis may seem to be smaller, and the dog will squat to urinate like a female. If the tumor is only in one testicle, the opposite one is likely to become quite small.

Testicular tumors are usually not malignant and tend to metastasize only late in their development, long past the time that you or your veterinarian should already have become aware of a tumor's existence. Castration removes the tumor and, if there has been no metastasis, *cures* your dog. All the associated symptoms will slowly disappear, and your dog will return to normal appearance within three to six months.

Many puppies grow into adulthood with either one or both testicles absent from the scrotum. It may be in front of the scrotum alongside the sheath (parasheath) or somewhere within the abdominal cavity (retained). This is often the result of an hereditary defect. Such an abnormally located testicle is more likely to develop tumors than one properly located within the scrotum. Since those in the abdomen remain sterile (cannot produce sperm cells), and those alongside the sheath also usually do not fully develop, many veterinarians recommend such dogs be castrated when young. This prevents the possibility of propagating the defect and precludes tumor development. The abdominally retained testicle is particularly dangerous, as tumors there can rarely be detected until advanced external symptoms appear. They are also more likely to be malignant and spread to nearby abdominal organs. The parasheath testicles are less potentially hazardous, as they can be seen and physically examined like scrotal testicles. Nevertheless, they do have a tendency to be malignant to a degree midway between scrotal and retained testicles.

Tumors of the Mammary Glands

Of all the benign and malignant tumors occurring in the female dog, breast tumors account for about one-half. Add to this a very definite age-related incidence, starting at six or seven, escalating rapidly to a peak between nine and twelve, and declining only slightly from there on, and I think you can appreciate the fact that your *intact* (unspayed) aging female dog is a very probable candidate for mammary tumors. Luckily about half of the many types of breast tumors found in dogs are benign and respond extremely well to surgical removal. Of course, this also means that the other half are malignant, often highly so, spreading rapidly to adjacent breasts, lymph nodes, lungs, and elsewhere.

Any one or more of the ten breasts your dog has can be affected by tumors, but the two pairs closest to the back legs are involved far more regularly than those farther forward. It therefore behooves you to do a home breast exam once a month, much as knowledgeable and cautious women do for themselves. Your family veterinarian will show you how to examine each breast for tiny lumps just beneath the skin or in the nipple. Be careful to handle the tissues gently, avoiding any rough squeezing or pressing.

Failure to detect small early abnormalities can result in slow growth between heat periods or rapid enlargement near, or during, estrus. Small tumors can become large inflamed or ulcerated masses slowly over weeks or months (for which there is *no* excuse) or rapidly within several days to a week or two (for which there is *little* excuse). Once ulcerated, such breasts become infected, making successful treatment far more difficult. Your dog's lungs will be X-rayed to detect any evidence of the tumor having spread. A negative report does not completely rule out metastasis, but is encouraging. A positive report of metastatic tumors in the lungs usually will preclude surgical therapy of the involved breast, unless it is mechanically troubling your dog.

All breast tumors should be surgically removed as soon as they are diagnosed, hopefully while they are still small. They are less likely to have spread if they turn out to be malignant, are easier to remove with less disfiguring, and may require a less extensive operation than larger tumors. Today, most veterinary surgeons will remove the affected breast, each adjacent unaffected breast and the related lymph nodes, all of which will be submitted to a pathologist. The pathologist will determine the type of tumor, whether it is benign or malignant, and whether or not it has metastasized. When the tumor is larger, or involves more than one breast, the surgeon will remove all the breasts on the same side, from armpit to groin, along with all the lymph nodes—a radical mastectomy. When tumors are present in breasts on both sides of the body, a two-stage operation may be recommended, with all the breasts on one side being removed at first, then the other side being removed several weeks later.

Following a mastectomy, your dog should be kept rather inactive, as even slow walking can cause a bit of discomfort. Watch for any signs of fluid accumulating under the skin or oozing from the incision, or your dog licking the incision excessively. These should be reported to your veterinarian. Skin sutures may be left in for two weeks or more, depending on the surgeon's preference and the type of suture material used. Soft, smooth, and clean bedding is important for your dog's comfort, even for an outdoor dog. In general, if there is no recurrence or growth at a new site within a year, you can consider your dog cured.

At nine and a half years of age, Kim, a large collie and shepherd mix, was in rather good general health except for a well-controlled kidney disorder she had had since she was seven. Following a normal heat period, she developed a small hard lump in one of her breasts, which grew to the size of an orange within ten days. Chest radiographs showed no signs of metastasis and surgery was advised. For carefully detailed reasons which I still don't understand to this day, the owner declined surgery and procrastinated for another month. By this time, small nodules were apparent in several other breasts on the same side and the original tumor was as big as a grapefruit. With a second X ray still showing no tumor spread in the lungs, the owner finally agreed to surgery. A radical mastectomy was done, removing all the breasts and lymph nodes on that side. Recovery and aftercare were without any special problems, but the pathologist's report showed the tumor to be a highly malignant type of mammary gland adenocarcinoma. Still, one year later there was no sign of any recurrence, and chest X rays were negative. At thirteen years of age, such was still the case until a summer vacation brought with it a fatal automobile injury.

Be the tumor malignant or benign, the prognosis is greatly improved if surgery is performed when it is small, well outlined, and not visibly spreading into surrounding tissues. If a report of cancer comes from the pathologist, your veterinarian may recommend chemotherapy after surgery. A dog with lung metastases and inoperable breast tumors may also derive some benefit for a short time from chemotherapy.

The occurrence of mammary tumors is definitely hormone related, and an intact female dog is at least one hundred times more likely to develop such tumors than a female spayed before her first heat period. Spaying an adult reduces the incidence but nowhere near the above figure. If your aged dog had an ovariohysterectomy as a puppy, you have little need to be concerned about breast tumors.

Male dogs are not excluded from developing breast tumors, although these are quite rare. All that has been said about the treatment of these tumors in the female applies to the male as well.

Pseudocyesis (False Pregnancy)

Your female dog was in heat about two months ago, and now she's behaving as if she were pregnant. Her breasts are somewhat enlarged and have a thin yellowish fluid or actual milk coming from them. She seems unusually nervous and excitable, can't settle down, and may even try to make a "nest." Finally you notice her carrying a shoe, toy, or other object around with her, much as she would a newborn puppy. But wait a minute, you say! She hasn't been near a male dog—she *can't* be pregnant! And she isn't. She is going through a false pregnancy.

When your bitch is in heat, a corpus luteum or yellow body is formed in the ovary, whether or not conception has taken place. During pregnancy, this corpus luteum remains active and functional, secreting the hormone, progesterone, until whelping time. In the nonpregnant bitch, the corpus usually degenerates in about a month. For reasons still not well understood, the corpus deteriorates much slower in some bitches, and its prolonged presence is believed to trigger the false pregnancy. Symptoms can vary from being hardly noticeable, through all those mentioned in the previous paragraph, to severe painful engorgement of the breasts with milk freely flowing from them.

Pseudocyesis occurs at all ages from the first puppy heat on. It may happen only once and never recur, but in most cases, once started, it tends to recur about two months after each, or most, of the successive heat periods. This can be a special problem in the older dog. The additional stress it produces can result in vomiting, diarrhea, self-nursing, inflammation and infection of one or more breasts, and loss of appetite. Dogs with chronic kidney disease may be stressed enough to precipitate a uremic crisis and renal failure (see Urinary System). Dogs with cardiac disease may develop potentially dangerous abnormal heart rhythms.

Mild to moderate cases will run their course in three to eight weeks, depending on how rapidly the corpus luteum degenerates, and require little treatment. The more severe cases will be helped by alternate hot and cold moist compresses on the swollen breasts to relieve the pain. Therapy with estrogens, testosterone, and, paradoxically, progesterone injections have all been effective to varying degrees in terminating the false pregnancy. The recently introduced "pill" for dogs, Ovaban®, can also be used to stop pseudocyesis. If fever or breast infection is present antibiotics will also be prescribed.

There is no hard evidence to prove it, but many veterinarians in companion animal practice are of the opinion that repeated false pregnancies, especially the severe ones, are likely to predispose your bitch to the eventual development of pyometra, a serious and hazardous uterine infection, discussed next. For that reason, as well as others already mentioned here and elsewhere, your family veterinarian may recommend an ovariohysterectomy for your dog.

Pyometra

Another problem of the female reproductive system related to prolonged activity of the corpus luteum, pyometra, is the accumulation of pus in the uterus. It is seen most frequently between three and six weeks after the dog has been in heat. Under the prolonged and repeated influence of progesterone from the corpus, the lining of the uterus becomes thickened, inflamed, and infected. Pus forms and may drain from the vulva as a gray, yellow-green, or brown discharge. The presence of this discharge and your dog's excessive licking at the vulva may be the only early indications you will have that your dog is ill. The chances of occurrence increase from middle age on and particularly in bitches who have not given birth for several years.

The presence of pyometra adversely affects other systems of the body including the liver, spleen, adrenal glands, and especially the kidneys. Increased thirst and increased urination (polydipsia and polyuria) are almost always present in pyometra, and vomiting, diarrhea, loss of appetite, and lethargy frequently accompany this disease. The uterine pus will discharge only if the cervix is open. Should it be completely or relatively closed, the pus accumulates in the uterus causing it to swell up like a balloon, distending the abdomen and putting pressure on all the other abdominal organs. Pressure is also brought aginst the diaphragm, thus reducing lung expansion and resulting in difficult breathing and poor air exchange. Such a *closed* pyometra can rapidly become an emergency situation as the adverse changes in each organ trigger problems in other organs. A self-perpetuating cascade of adversity develops which quickly produces a state of unhealth incompatible with the continuation of life.

Your veterinarian will many times be able to feel the enlarged uterus through the abdominal wall, even if the pus is discharging. Blood tests show a significant elevation in white blood cells; the result of the body's attempt to fight the infection, and your dog will usually have a fever. Before deciding on a course of action, your veterinarian will also perform certain kidney function tests and may radiograph the abdomen in order to confirm the diagnosis, rule out the remote possibility of an abnormal but real pregnancy, and detect the presence of any other complicating intra-abdominal disorders.

The treatment of choice is an ovariohysterectomy, performed as quickly as your dog's overall state of health will permit. The pus filled, infected uterus, as well as both ovaries and their ligaments, are completely removed. This is a serious operation, not only because of the presence of all that pus in the uterus, but because of the deleterious effect pyometra has on the kidneys, liver, and other organs. In the geriatric dog complications are not uncommon. Your veterinarian will have anticipated some of these from the results of the presurgical examination and will be better able to handle them, if they develop, or even totally prevent their occurrence. In-hospital care will be longer than that following a normal "spay," and frequent return visits to check kidney and liver function may be needed in the older dog.

When operated early, before the poisonous pus has further damaged already weakened liver and kidneys, the success rate is high. So much so that owners of such dogs frequently tell me "she's acting like a puppy again" or "she's like a new dog." The improvement is that obvious. Like it was with Dolly, a terrier who developed pyometra when she was eleven and a half, had a successful ovariohysterectomy done, and lived to be almost eighteen.

Jeannie's owner was sure her pet had diabetes when this twelve-year-old Afghan hound started drinking excessively. Upon examination and X ray, however, we were able to diagnose pyometra. A complete presurgical exam was done, and the operation performed later that same day. Except for a brief flare-up of a previously stabilized erratic heartbeat, which was brought under control rather quickly, the reovery went smoothly, and Jeannie was home in a few days acting like the proverbial puppy. The owner was so pleased, he requested I immediately remove four small skin tumors that I had been after him to have operated since the dog was nine. We did remove them, but not until Jeannie had some more time to get fully over her ovariohysterectomy.

The open cervix, draining pyometra can *sometimes* be successfully treated by a medical, rather than surgical, approach. However, the chance of recurrence following subsequent heat periods is high. Yet it can be the preferable course in a very old dog whose life expectancy at the time might only be a year or two. It may also be the choice for the dog with marginally stabilized kidney or cardiac disease which would drastically raise the anesthetic and surgical risks. Antibiotics and several different hormones have been used, along with mechanically flushing out the uterus. Your veterinarian will use whatever methods work best in his hands, but keep in mind that medical treatment is only temporary at best, and the problem is very likely to recur.

Mismating (Accidental Breeding)

The undesired and accidental breeding of a female dog can be a distressing incident for any owner. But for you, the owner of an aging female, such an event can be fraught with potential difficulties irrespective of "what shall I do with the puppies?" The stresses of pregnancy can precipitate cardiovascular, kidney, musculoskeletal, and other problems and should be avoided. The best prevention, short of an ovariohysterectomy, is never to let your dog off the leash when she is in heat. While the symptoms may not be as prominent as in younger years, she will be in heat.

Should an accidental breeding take place in spite of your diligent precautions, pregnancy may still be prevented if you act promptly. Estrogens administered by your veterinarian by injection within the first twenty-four to forty-eight hours will generally prevent the implantation of any fertilized eggs into the uterine wall. It will also prolong the heat period and the length of time your bitch will continue to attract male dogs! Take care you don't allow another accidental breeding.

Once implantation has occurred and pregnancy is established, the use of estrogens, as above, has little value and may be fraught with danger. Surgical removal of the ovaries will terminate the pregnancy and, while not often done, is a possible approach. In most cases, if surgery is decided upon, an ovariohysterectomy will be done, thus removing the fetuses as well as the source of potential future problems. As of the present writing, there is no safe and effective medical treatment to induce an abortion in the female dog.

6
The Cardiovascular System

The normal canine heart beats between seventy and one hundred sixty times a minute, every minute of the day, every day of the year, with the faster rates occurring in the smaller breeds and the slower rates in the larger ones. If we take one hundred twenty as an "average rate" for all breeds, that average heart will have made slightly more than *631 million* contractions by the time your dog is ten years old! Is it any wonder that almost one-fourth of all dogs have some kind of heart abnormality by the time they reach that age? Yet embolism (blood clot) of the heart's own blood vessels, which causes a "heart attack" in people, is not at all common in dogs.

In the geriatric canine most heart disease results either from malfunctioning of the heart valves or a disturbance in the transmission of the heart impulse from the upper (atria) to the lower (ventricles) heart chambers. Each generally develops rather slowly over several years before causing noticeable signs of disease, although an occasional dog can become ill in only a matter of weeks. Both of these abnormalities can eventually result in congestive heart failure.

Diagnosing Heart Disease

There are several general symptoms which tend to be suggestive of heart disease. A recurrent deep cough, especially at night and upon awakening, tiring very quickly, and a distended abdomen accompanied by labored breathing are prime examples. These are not symptoms specific just to heart disease, and if your dog has any of them, they could just as easily be caused by noncardiac disorders. The diagnosis of heart disease is arrived at by means of a three-part diagnostic workup consisting of auscultation of the heart and lungs (listening with a stethoscope), radiographs of the heart and lungs, and an electrocardiogram or ECG. It is rare that one of these procedures alone will give a definitive diagnosis, as each gathers a different type of information. Collectively they do give a rather clear picture of what is happening to the heart.

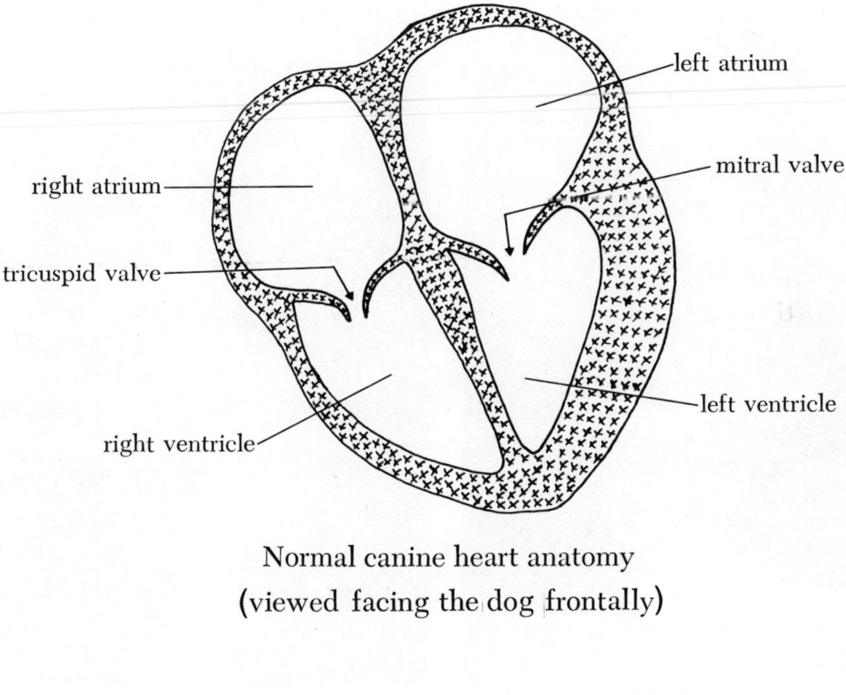

Normal canine heart anatomy
(viewed facing the dog frontally)

AUSCULTATION

Your family veterinarian will listen to your dog's heart and lungs with a stethoscope to determine the regularity, rate, duration, and quality of each phase of the heartbeat. He will also listen for any abnormal heart sounds, usually referred to as heart murmurs. Areas of increased or decreased sounds in the lungs will be noted at this time.

RADIOGRAPHS

At least two X rays of your dog's heart and lungs will be taken, one view from the side and the other view from the front (underside) of the chest. Together they give a sort of three-dimensional picture of these organs. Changes in the shape of the heart and major blood vessels, as well as in the structure of the lungs, can indicate where the cardiac disorder actually is located.

Radiographs of normal and abnormal hearts. Note the difference in the shape of the heart. Both views are from the underside of the chest.

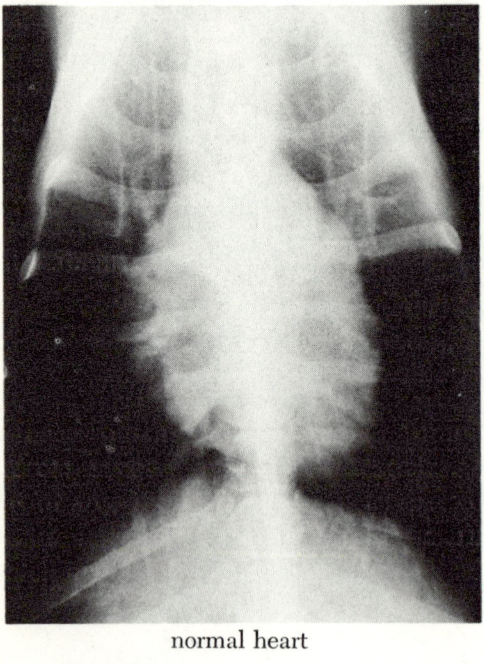

normal heart

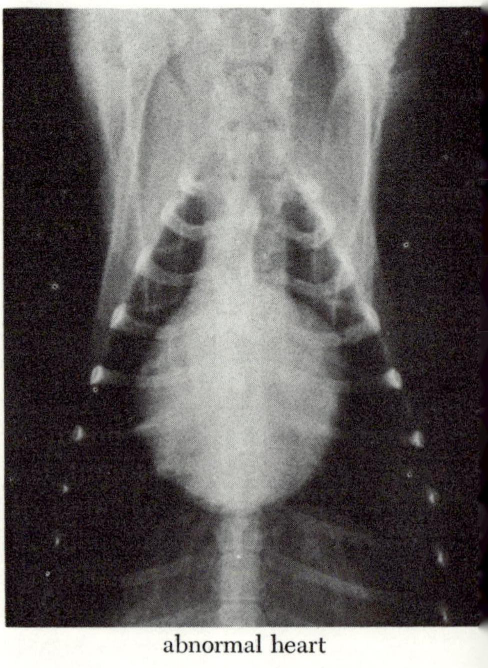

abnormal heart

ELECTROCARDIOGRAM

This diagnostic procedure is performed on your dog essentially the same way it would be done on you. The only major difference is, that instead of the end of each cable being wrapped around your wrists and ankles, they are attached to your dog's elbows and stifles by small clips which cause no discomfort. One other difference is that your physician can expect you to lie motionless on your back, while your dog will have to be held on his side, and he may or may not remain still. There is no pain or discomfort associated with the making of an ECG tracing, and *no* electricity passes into your dog. However, many dogs just don't like to lie quietly on their side for the two or three minutes it takes to make such a tracing.

The electrocardiogram records the electrical output—discharge and recharge—of the myriad of muscle fibers which make up the heart muscle. These electrical changes normally occur in a very definite order and at predictable time intervals. Changes in the order or intervals indicate heart abnormalities and may exist even when auscultation is normal and radiographs show no changes.

An electrocardiogram is able to indicate heart rate, regular or irregular rhythm, enlargement of any of the four heart chambers, as well as abnormal heart rhythm sequences or arrhythmias. Reading and interpreting an ECG takes skill and experience; but the next time your veterinarian shows you your dog's electrocardiogram and speaks of wide P waves, tall QRS complexes, or points to a ventricular premature contraction, you will be better able to understand him. Refer to the ECG tracing shown on page 126 as you read along.

Each normal canine heartbeat produces an ECG tracing like that shown at 1. The various deflections or "waves" are named with the letters P through T as marked. In 2 the tall P wave indicates enlargement of the right atrium; the wide P wave in 3 denotes enlargement of the left atrium. Left ventricular enlargement is shown by the wider and very tall R wave in 4. Enlargement of the right ventricle usually produces a deep S wave and a wide QRS complex as in 5. An increase or decrease in the distances between the P wave, QRS complex, and T wave denotes abnormal

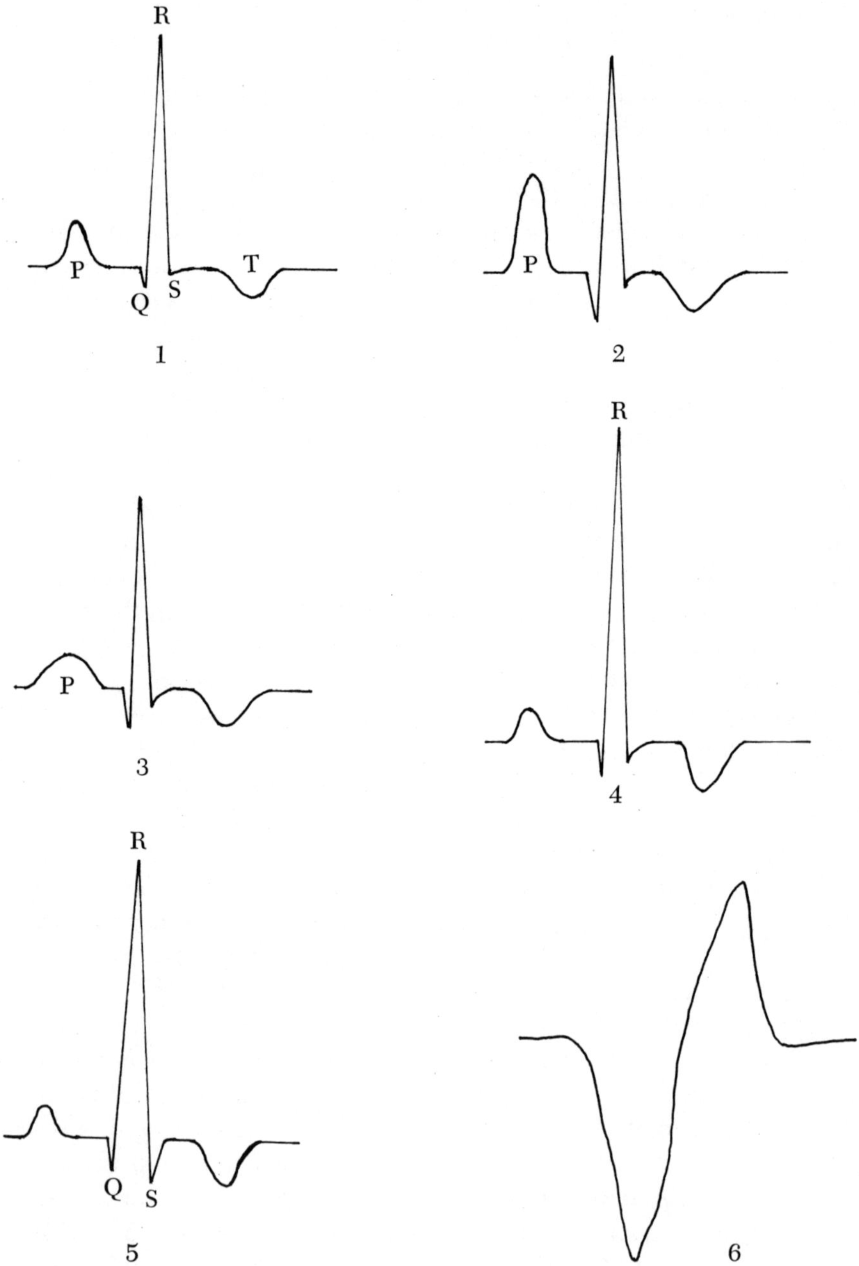

Anatomy of an electrocardiogram.

rhythms, as does the premature contraction of the ventricles shown in 6. Of course you realize these illustrations are very much simplified and that there is a wide variety of combinations of heart abnormalities which can occur in aging dogs. At least now those squiggles on a long piece of graphlike paper will have some meaning for you.

Let me, at this point, clarify a seeming abnormality in dogs which often upsets an owner. The rhythm of the human heart is normally very regular whereas that of a dog is *rarely ever* regular when at rest. The dog's heart will beat several times in regular rhythm, then slow as if a beat or two were being skipped, only to speed up again to the original or near original rhythm. This is called *sinus arrhythmia* and is normal in the resting dog. In fact, should your dog exhibit a perfectly regular rhythm while at rest, he may very well have some type of heart disease. When he is running or is excited, however, the beat does become quite regular.

Sometimes the collective data obtained by auscultation, X rays, and ECG is still not adequate to make a definitive diagnosis. In these cases, a cardiac catheterization may be done. Under general anesthesia, a very narrow tube is put into one of the major blood vessels leading to the heart. It is then passed into whichever part of the heart is suspected of being abnormal. A dye which shows on X rays is then injected through the tube into the heart, and a series of radiographs are taken in rapid succession. The speed and direction of dye movement through the heart helps pinpoint the disorder. This procedure is most useful in diagnosing congenital heart disorders in the young dog but is occasionally indicated in aged-dog heart disease.

Chronic Heart Valve Disease

During the relaxing phase of each heartbeat, blood flows from the atria into the ventricles through valves which then close as the heart begins its contraction phase. It is during this second phase that blood is pumped to the lungs and, via the aorta, to all other parts of the body. The valve on the left side is called the mitral and the one on the right side, the tricuspid valve. Starting sometimes as early as three or four years old, these valves *slowly* and *pro-*

gressively become thickened, develop lumps on their edges and may actually shrink in size. During cardiac contraction, these misshapen valves cannot tightly close to prevent the backflow of blood into the atria and are, in effect, leaky valves. The inappropriate backflow of blood from the ventricle to the atrium usually produces an audible sound or murmur which can be heard with a stethoscope.

As the next relaxation phase takes place this ventricular blood, now in the atrium, again flows into the ventricle along with the new blood arriving from the atrium. This continuing increase in the volume of blood entering the ventricle causes that chamber to dilate in order to make room for the extra blood. Unfortunately, this tends to pull the edges of the heart valves even further apart. As the chamber enlarges, it becomes increasingly difficult for the stretched heart muscle to contract with adequate force, so the heart's muscular wall undergoes hypertrophy and becomes thicker and thicker. The combination of dilatation and hypertrophy makes the heart physically bigger but not necessarily more effective in performing its intended job of pumping blood. The cause of chronic heart valve disease is still unknown, although many theoretical explanations have been evolved. Also for as yet unknown reasons, there seems to be a somewhat higher incidence among toy and small dogs.

The early stage of heart valve abnormality usually produces no outward signs, the dog appearing to be quite normal. Yet with diligent use of his stethoscope, your veterinarian may be able to hear a barely audible murmur as he gives your dog her annual examination. When the disease progresses, which it may not do for months or years, the valves leak more, the heart enlarges, and a number of characteristic, but not necessarily pathognomonic symptoms begin to appear. Perhaps the most noticeable is a deep cough most evident at night or in the early morning hours, which later also occurs during waking hours and can be triggered by excitement, pulling on a leash, or even eating or drinking. Increasing lung congestion causes periods of labored breathing which may manifest itself by your dog's reluctance to lie down, a position in which breathing often can become more difficult. The resultant restlessness, occurring during the day as well, is most apparent at night, when your dog's pacing is likely to wake you up. Fluid ac-

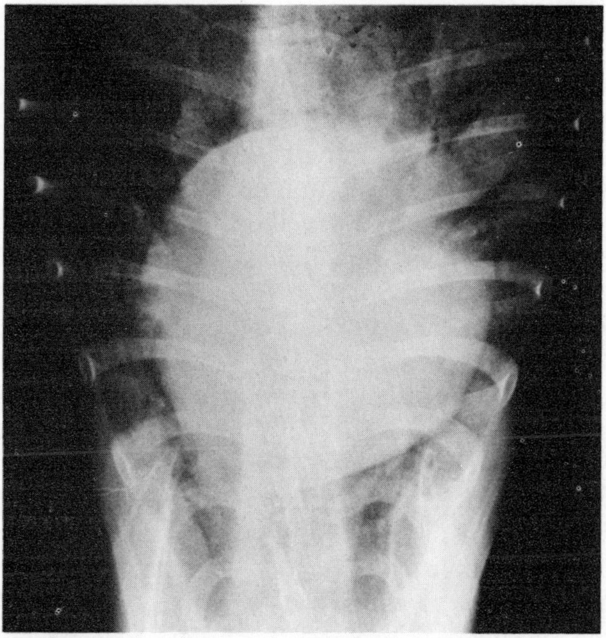

Radiograph of an enlarged heart. Note the almost circular shape, compared to the normal heart shown on page 124.

cumulating in the abdomen can cause a pot belly, and the legs and feet may be swollen. Weakness, reduced appetite, occasional vomiting or diarrhea, and changes in the amount or frequency of urination are other symptoms which should alert you.

A complete physical exam is essential, even though the history and symptoms pretty much point to heart disease, in order to rule out "look alike" disorders and assess kidney and liver function, both of which are intimately related to adequate heart function. X rays of the chest will detect changes in the size and shape of the heart in addition to showing fluid or other changes in the lungs. An electrocardiogram will confirm the diagnosis and provide other information on the physiological state of your dog's heart.

Except for complete replacement by prosthetic (artificial) valves, there is no cure for chronic heart valve disease. Medical treatment is directed at controlling the adverse symptoms and improving cardiac function. Such control and improvement sometimes last only a few weeks but more often are successful for many months up to one or two years, and once in a while, even longer.

Since the cause is unknown at present, nothing can be done to stop further progressive damage to the valves.

Rest and restriction of activity are important to reduce the heart's work load. Exercise, unnecessary running or walking, stair climbing, jumping, and the like should be limited or totally stopped, as your veterinarian indicates. The restriction will be determined by the severity of the disease process and may change from time to time as the heart improves or declines. It can be difficult to do this with some of the more active breeds, and it will take a conscious, concerted effort on your part to accomplish what is required. Let's face it, you cannot put your dog to bed the way you would yourself in a similar condition. But you know your dog well enough after all these years, that by anticipating and keeping a step ahead of his next move, you can help him to avoid most of the undesirable activities.

Medications fall into three functional areas. Bronchodilators enlarge the tubular passages of the lungs, making it easier to breathe and reducing some of the coughing. Diuretics remove fluid from the lungs, abdomen, and swollen legs through the kidneys; again, improving respiration and physical comfort. Digitalis-like drugs improve heart muscle strength and slow the heart rate, enabling that organ to pump blood more efficiently. There are a number of different drugs available in each of these groups, and it may be necessary during long-term therapy to change from one to another within a group. These three types of medication may, at any given time, be used alone or in combination with any of the others. Again, such combinations may have to be changed from time to time as your dog's response or lack of it indicates.

As the ailing heart pumps poorly, the blood pressure flowing through the kidneys is reduced, and several complex changes occur in these organs. The normal kidney excretes any excess sodium there may be in the body, but in advancing heart disease this excretion is diminished, sodium levels begin to rise and fluid is retained, accumulating in the lungs, abdomen, and legs. Although not needed for every heart patient, many such affected dogs do benefit from a low sodium diet. This is available, commercially prepared, and can be prescribed by your doctor. Whether in dry or canned form, however, it is not very palatable, and getting an older dog to eat it can frequently be a chore. By adding water to it, you improve the texture and palatability considerably. Always start by mixing one or two teaspoonfuls of the heart diet with your dog's regular food. Once he accepts it, gradually increase the amount of heart diet over a week or two, decreasing the regular diet proportionately until it is eliminated. Most dogs will eat it if you persist. When needed, these commercial diets are probably the best.

If you are willing to prepare a special diet for your dog, as I'm sure you are, you can use the following list of foods to choose from. Your veterinarian will guide you as to specific amounts in order to supply adequate, but not excessive, calories and protein. She may also have other food suggestions, as this list is far from complete.

Permitted	*Not Permitted*
Pork, *fresh*	Bacon or ham
Lamb, *fresh*	Sausage or lunch meats
Beef, *fresh*	Beef liver, heart or kidney
Veal, *fresh*	Baby food meats, unless salt free
Chicken, white meat, *fresh*	Chicken, dark meat
Rabbit, *fresh*	Canned or processed meats
Fish, *fresh water*	All shellfish
Eggs, *yolk only*	Egg whites
Milk, *low sodium*	All other dairy products including ice cream and yogurt
Margarine, *unsalted*	
Most vegetables, *fresh*	All canned vegetables
Spaghetti and macaroni	Bread
Rice and potato	Cake and cookies
Cereals, *cooked*	Cereals, *dry*
Fruit, *fresh*	Fruit, *dried*
Sugar	Candy
Honey	Molasses
Garlic	Garlic salt
Onion powder	Onion salt
Pepper	Mustard

The initial therapy of your cardiac dog may be done on an outpatient basis if the symptoms are mild. With advanced symptoms, and particularly if the digitalis drugs are used, your dog will probably be hospitalized until the symptoms are relieved and a maintenance dose of each drug has been established. If your dog is one of those who does not do well in strange surroundings, your veterinarian will treat even some advanced cases as out-patients in order to avoid the extra stress. Either way, it is desirable to monitor the heart's response with frequent electrocardiograms until adequate control of the heart is secured. Frequent testing of blood sodium and potassium levels may also have to be done. Even if your dog remains symptom free, he should be examined at least once every three months.

Open-Heart Surgery

Virtually all methods and techniques of performing surgery within the heart that are used today in human medicine were first developed experimentally on dogs. It should therefore follow that open-heart surgery is readily available to the canine cardiac patient. Not quite so. Because canine red blood cells are more fragile and easily damaged by the mechanical movement inherent in these operations than are human red cells, the procedure is much more complicated. The extensive and elaborate equipment specially needed for these operations is to be found only in colleges of human medicine and their hospitals, a few veterinary colleges, and some heart disease research centers. Relatively few veterinary surgeons are trained in such techniques, and the overall costs of the time-consuming surgery, postoperative care, and hospitalization would probably be prohibitive for most dog owners.

Open-heart surgery has its greatest usefulness in the correction of congenital or early developmental cardiac defects. In the aging dog, it could be of value for those with chronic heart valve disease. A few such dogs have successfully had those valves replaced with prosthetic ones. If your dog could be helped by such an operation, and you have the means to pursue it, your family veterinarian can refer you to the nearest institution where both properly trained veterinary surgeons and the necessary equipment are available.

Cardiac Arrhythmia

Listen to your dog's heartbeat, or put your fingers on her chest wall to feel it. Do it right now, if possible. "The beat isn't steady! Every few beats it skips one! What's wrong with my dog?" Perhaps nothing at all. What you are hearing or feeling is called *sinus arrhythmia* and is a normal arrhythmia in dogs. It is due to the shape of their chest and their breathing patterns. Any change in the rate or regularity of the heartbeat is called an arrhythmia. If the heart beats too fast (tachycardia), there is not enough time for it to fill properly during relaxation, and less blood is pumped out when it contracts. Bradycardia (very slow heartbeat) is less dangerous, but if extreme, it too can result in insufficient blood being pumped around the body, and your dog will become lethargic. Alterations in the normal production of the heart's electrical impulse or changes in its transmission through the heart, or both, can cause all kinds of arrhythmias.

Some few abnormal rhythms can be detected by your veterinarian by listening to the heart and taking the pulse in a rear leg artery at the same time. But the accurate diagnosis of the particular type of arrhythmia, and where it originates from, requires an electrocardiogram. Symptoms will vary from one type to another but can include periodic or continuous weakness, fainting or sudden collapse, labored breathing, and fluid in the abdomen. It is also quite possible that there may be no external signs in some of the early arrhythmic stages.

Abnormal heart rhythms can occur independently of, or in conjunction with, chronic valve or other heart disease. There are many drugs used to treat arrhythmias. They speed up or slow down the heart rate and either enhance or retard electrical impulse transmission. Such drugs usually have to be given indefinitely and must initially be frequently monitored with electrocardiograms.

Certain types of abnormally slow heart rhythms do not respond well to medical therapy or else respond initially and then fail. For such dogs an artificial heart pacemaker can be put in place to stimulate the diseased heart electrically to beat at a proper rate. The dog will need periodic follow-up to be sure the unit continues to function correctly. Most units available today will operate satisfactorily for from eighteen months up to five years, before their batteries need replacement. New developments in battery manufacture will undoubtedly extend their life well beyond that. Pacemakers for humans were experimentally developed in dogs, so their use is certainly readily applicable to those older dogs whose cardiac disease is treatable with pacemaker therapy.

The major cost of such an operation is that of the pacemaker itself, which usually exceeds twelve hundred dollars. In recent years, veterinarians who do this advanced cardiac surgery have been able to obtain pacemakers previously used in people at substantially lower cost. Despite being "second hand," once fitted with new batteries, they function quite well.

Congestive Heart Failure

In the majority of aging dogs, chronic heart valve disease, dilatation, hypertrophy, and many arrhythmias lead eventually to congestive heart failure. Having succeeded for variable lengths of time in making up for the heart's decreased ability effectively to pump enough oxygen-laden blood throughout the body, the heart begins to lose its capacity to compensate. Any or all prior cardiac symptoms can return and will usually be more exaggerated. Labored breathing and coughing even while resting, pulmonary and pleural effusions (see Respiratory System), bluish-red or darker gums and tongue, weakness, ascites (abdominal fluid), and fainting are the signs most commonly observed. Just about any kind of movement or activity will make the symptoms worse and cause total collapse.

The appearance of the above-noted symptoms in your cardiac dog already is, or will rapidly become, an emergency situation. Immediately phone your veterinarian, and take your dog to her hospital, regardless of the hour! She will give you instructions how to move your dog, but, in general, these are basics. Move gently but quickly, trying not to alarm your dog. Wrap him in a blanket with his head exposed, supporting him under the front and back legs, rather than the chest or abdomen. With rare exceptions, your dog will be hospitalized and be given oxygen to alleviate the breathing distress. Anxious and frightened because of his difficulties, he will probably be given a mild sedative to relax him. Digitalislike drugs to slow, but strengthen, the heart and intravenous diuretics for rapid removal of the excess body fluids will be administered. In extreme ascites, some of the abdominal fluid will be withdrawn with a syringe and needle. It may even be necessary to remove some of your dog's blood in order quickly to reduce the heart's work load. As your dog shows some improvement, other medications will also be indicated. X rays, electrocardiograms, and certain blood tests may have to be done frequently during the first twenty-four to forty-eight hours of this intensive treatment.

Once stabilized, your dog will be sent home on one of the digitalis drugs, diuretics, a low salt diet, and possibly bronchodilators and a cough suppressant. Antiarrhythmic medications will also be prescribed if the congestive heart failure was accompanied or caused by an abnormal rhythm.

A word of caution about the digitalis-related drugs. They tend to accumulate in the body, although slowly. Modern forms are somewhat safer than the older ones, but the margin of safety between the effective dose and a dangerous dose can still be very narrow. Measure the prescribed dose very carefully, whether liquid or tablet, and do not exceed it. Should the accumulated level become excessive *most* dogs will start to vomit before the heart is endangered. In that event, assuming there is no other likely reason to account for the vomiting, skip the next dose of the drug, and contact your veterinarian for further instructions.

Quiet and rest for the remainder of your dog's life are essential, but you will be advised when, and to what limited extent, slow walking can be permitted.

Follow-up exams should be done within a week or two of discharge from the hospital and at regular intervals thereafter. Acute recurrences of the symptoms of congestive heart failure can and do take place with a disturbing frequency despite all known therapy. When your dog's heart has reached this stage of disorder, his life expectancy is significantly reduced. He can be made quite comfortable and happy, but treatment neither cures nor improves the underlying condition. Nor can it effectively stop further deterioration, so that "time left" is often only from six months to a year.

Certain kinds of heart disease develop secondary to uremia and other kidney disorders or from severe anemia. Cardiac therapy must be preceded or accompanied by treatment of the underlying cause. Ascites, so "characteristic" of congestive heart failure, is also caused by severe liver disease and must not be assumed to be a sign of a bad heart.

Early heart disease was diagnosed during her annual geriatric exam when Gambi was seven and a half. Conservative therapy kept this Doberman mix alert, symptom free, and relatively active for the following seven years, despite the progressive nature of her heart ailment. Her death at fourteen and a half years of age was due to inoperable lung cancer and unrelated to her cardiac problem.

Winston is a tough little pug who probably would not have lived past seven years, had he been born twenty-five or thirty years ago. He is now twelve and gives every indication that he plans on being around for quite a while, in spite of his chronic heart disease. During an examination for an acute gastro-intestinal upset when he was six, an abnormal heart rhythm was discovered. An electrocardiogram showed the arrhythmia to be secondary to the intestinal disorder, and not a primary heart problem. However, other information from the ECG and chest X rays indicated early enlargement of both ventricles and the left atrium. No cardiac therapy was needed, as the dog was quite well and symptom-free once the digestive disturbance was resolved, and the heart remained stable for almost two years.

After that period, a slight left-side heart murmur which had not been audible previously was heard during a regular checkup. Changes in the ECG and X rays confirmed that Winston's heart was slowly enlarging, and the mitral valve was not closing completely. But Winston didn't know from ECG's or X rays and didn't know there was anything wrong with his heart. He continued to behave like a perfectly healthy dog, showing none of the symptoms I would have expected. However, almost two years later, at the age of nine and a half, he suddenly started slowing down, breathing very heavily, and coughing during much of the night as well as pacing restlessly. Examination showed the ventricles to be even larger, and there were changes in the heart beat.

Fluid sounds could be heard in both lungs as Winston was having his first serious bout of chronic heart valve disease. He was started on bronchodilators along with one of the digitalis drugs and responded quite well. So well, in fact, that when he came back for a checkup, three days after he had been stabilized, his owner said, "He feels so good he's just like a puppy again."

Three months later, Winston developed a temporary sensitivity to the digitalis drug, began to vomit, and have all kinds of electrocardiographic abnormalities. The drug was discontinued for twenty-four hours and then reinstituted at a lower dosage. He was fine for a month but started to cough again. The drug was increased slightly without any side effects, and he was as "good as new" within a week.

For another year and a half, Winston's heart remained stable, both in terms of being relatively symptom-free and no further changes on X rays or ECG's. Then the coughing began again, accompanied this time by general weakness, increased thirst and increased urination. The digitalis drug dose was increased slightly more, diuretics were given, and he was put on a low-salt diet and a potassium supplement. Once more, this indomitable pug bounced right back, but this time he seems to have learned to read the X rays and ECG, and is behaving accordingly. Although he is less active and at twelve is suddenly showing his age for the first time, he nevertheless continues to do well at this writing.

Emergency Cardiac Massage

At some point during the course of your dog's life, if she has cardiac disease, her heart may actually stop beating. Prompt action by you *might* be able to start it again and save her life, but you have only six minutes in which to succeed. Lack of blood and oxygen for longer than that will produce irreversible brain damage.

Lay your dog on her right side, on the floor or other hard surface. Place the palm of your right hand on the back of your left hand. Now put the palm of your left hand, with the right hand on top of it, on her chest wall just behind her elbow. With both hands, press firmly and sharply down on the chest wall; hold momentarily and release. The compression time should be twice as long as the release period. This cycle should be repeated approximately sixty times a minutes. In barrel-chested breeds, lay the dog on her back and press straight down on the sternum (breastbone), using your hands in the same arrangement. If there is someone else to help you, have them open your dog's mouth, wipe out any saliva or vomited food, pull the tongue forward, and start mouth to mouth resuscitation at a rate of twenty to thirty times a minute. Should you be alone you must do this yourself. Every fifth time you press on the chest wall, stop and blow strongly into your dog's mouth, watching to be certain the chest rises as your breath expands her lungs. Then go back to the cardiac massage. It is not easy to do this alone, but you have no choice.

Mouth to mouth resuscitation itself may not be easy either, due to the varying shapes and sizes of mouth found in the more than one hundred twenty-five breeds of dog. In general, if your dog's mouth is big enough to permit doing so, place your mouth *inside* hers. Otherwise place your mouth *over* hers and her nose. In either case, her tongue must be pulled forward and out to one side, and held there with your fingers in order to keep the entrance to the trachea (windpipe) open. It is rarely possible nor is it desirable to get an airtight seal, what with the mismatched mouth contours and the tongue protruding from one side. In the smaller breeds this will prevent you from overinflating the lungs but in the larger breeds you'll have to blow with considerable effort to start the lungs expanding. In either case stop blowing as soon as you can see the chest wall rise.

Both external cardiac massage and artificial respiration are best learned by demonstration and practice, rather than by reading about them. Ask your veterinarian to show you how to do these life saving measures on *your* dog.

Continue this heart massage and artificial respiration until you can feel the heart beating again, she starts breathing, and the blue-gray color of her tongue and gums changes to pink. Keep her absolutely quiet and watch her carefully as the heart may stop again. Once breathing starts, she will benefit from oxygen if you have an emergency tank available. Phone your veterinarian and carefully follow his directions for transporting your dog to his clinic where she will receive further treatment to stabilize the heart and correct the severe imbalances—in body salt, potassium, and other chemicals—which occurred during the time her heart wasn't beating.

Tumors

Tumors *in* the canine heart are rare. There is, however, a commoner tumor which develops just outside the heart, at its base, and is known as an aortic body tumor or heart base tumor. It is found mostly in older male brachycephalic dogs (those with characteristically pushed-in faces), especially English bulldogs, boxers, and Boston terriers. These tumors are slow-growing but eventually put pressure on the heart and the large blood vessels which come out at the base of the heart, producing symptoms similar to those of congestive heart failure. Unfortunately, by the time these symptoms develop, the tumor has so invaded surrounding tissue as to make surgical removal virtually impossible. Your veterinarian will prescribe medications to symptomatically treat and sustain heart function for as long as possible.

Heartworm Disease

Once considered to be limited in the United States to the southern part of the country, canine heartworm disease has spread rapidly during the past decade. There have been at least a few cases reported from just about every state in the Union, and the disease has become widespread over most of the eastern half of the country, from south to north, and on up into many parts of Canada (see the accompanying map). It is also a worldwide disease occurring in Mexico, Central America, the coastal countries of South America and Africa, southern Europe, southeast Asia, coastal Australia, eastern China, and southern Japan.

The adult heartworm lives, as its name implies, within the heart—in the right atrium and ventricle as well as in the large blood vessels which enter and leave those chambers. These worms range in length from six to about fourteen inches, and their presence interferes with the flow of blood through, and out of, the heart to the lungs.

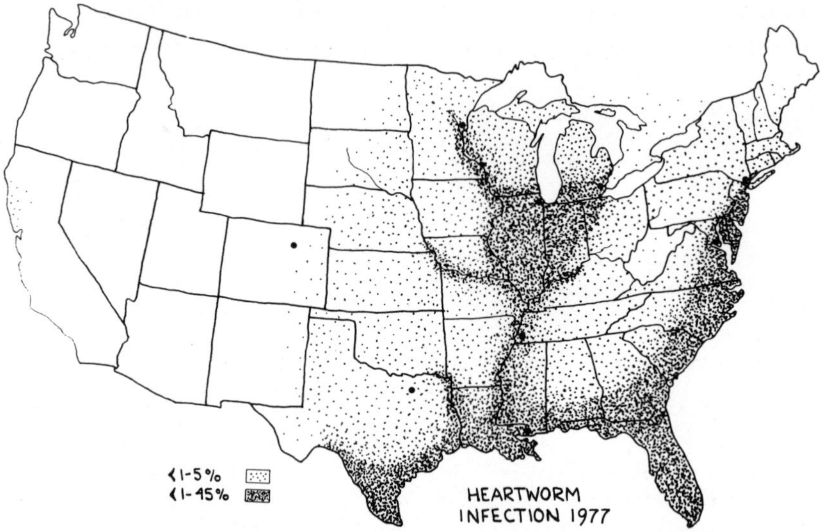

Incidence of canine heartworm infection in the United States in 1977. *Courtesy of The American Heartworm Society.*

Although this is a transmissible disease, it is not contagious from dog to dog. As with intestinal tapeworms, there must be an intermediate host. In the case of the heartworm, known as *Dirofilaria immitis*, that host is a mosquito; but there are dozens of different kinds of mosquitoes which can be an effective host. One reason believed to account for the recent rapid spread of this disease is that more varieties of these flying insects, living in colder climates, have become satisfactory intermediate hosts. Short-coated dogs are at a much higher risk than those with longer hair coats, as are outdoor dogs—particularly those who sleep outdoors—compared to house dogs.

It is important to understand the life cycle of the heartworm in order to fully appreciate the special hazard it holds for the aging dog. Adult worms in your dog's heart, which can live for up to five years, breed, and produce active microscopic-sized babies called microfilaria, which move quickly into the circulating blood throughout the body. A mosquito bites your dog and in the process drinks some of the infected blood. The microfilaria inside the mosquito develop through several growth stages to become infective larvae in approximately two weeks. The mosquito is not injured in any way by this growth, and when it subsequently bites a healthy dog's skin, these larvae are passed into that dog. They migrate under the skin for about three months, all the while undergoing further development into young adults, which takes another two or three months to migrate through the body to the heart where, after mating, the cycle begins again.

Any given dog may harbor as few as a single parasite or as many as two or three *hundred* adult worms. As the space in the heart gets crowded, many of the worms migrate into the pulmonary artery going to the lungs and the vena cava veins returning blood from the rest of the body, especially from the liver. They not only interfere with blood flow but can prevent the heart valves from adequately opening or closing, cause right-side heart enlargement, completely plug up small blood vessels in the lungs, and seriously damage the liver and kidneys. It should now be apparent why a disease which can affect dogs from the moment they are born and throughout life is included in this book. Heartworm disease is a hazard to life at any age but is a special danger to the aging dog who may already have heart, lung, kidney, or liver disease from other causes.

Like many serious diseases of dogs, this one develops slowly and often shows no outward signs until it is quite advanced, making the treatment more dangerous. The only chance for early diagnosis is to find the microfilaria in a blood sample while your dog is still symptom-free. For this reason, such a test should be included in your dog's annual geriatric exam, even in areas where the disease is presently rare. Heartworm disease is spreading rapidly, and what is today's heartworm-free area may be tomorrow's disease-laden area. The test is quick, painless and will detect about eighty-five percent of infected dogs. For the other fifteen percent, diagnosis can be a problem, requiring chest X rays which can show an enlarged right heart and distended or twisted lung arteries. An electrocardiogram and other laboratory tests are also useful to confirm an otherwise equivocal diagnosis of heartworm disease. Some of the symptoms of advanced disease are shortness of breath, coughing, sudden tiring or collapsing during or after exercise, and sometimes ascites. Obviously, all can be signs of another disease as well.

With our newer knowledge of how heartworms produce disease

and our increased ability to keep dogs healthier as they age, the treatment of this disease is no longer the very dangerous and often lethal therapy it was only twenty years ago, even though most of the same medications are still being used. Nevertheless, blood and urine tests to assess the functional status of the liver, kidneys, and other organs accurately, must be done before treatment is started and repeated many times during and after treatment. Your dog will be hospitalized during the first phase of therapy, which consists of a series of injections of an arsenic drug into the bloodstream. Yes, you read it correctly—arsenic! This drug kills the adult worms, and, if there are no adverse reactions, you will have your dog home in three or four days. Some dogs do have bad reactions, and the injections have to be delayed or stopped altogether. Rarely, a dog may die but this is unusual today.

The first six weeks after treatment are the most critical and, if not properly tended to, can result in serious illness and death. As the adult worms die they disintegrate and slowly pass out of the heart and large blood vessels into the tiny vessels of the lungs, where the body's defense systems seal them off. If this process goes on slowly, the slight loss of tiny portions of the lungs and the inflammation resulting from the dead worms being sealed off can successfully be adjusted to by the dog's body. On the other hand, if large numbers of dead worms move rapidly, as can occur with excitement and exercise, dangerous episodes of coughing and difficult breathing will occur and serious complications result. Your cooperation in keeping your dog as quiet and inactive as possible is the key to a successful outcome. Apartment-house dogs should avoid stairs; outdoor dogs should be confined to a leash. You must anticipate all things which might cause excitement and avoid them. During the first or second week after treatment, even a quiet dog may cough some and have a fever. This is very common. Your veterinarian will give you medication to control it and make your dog more comfortable.

At the end of six weeks, assuming all reactions have disappeared, an oral medication is given to get rid of the microfilaria (remember, the arsenic killed only the adults). It is given for one week or until blood tests show the microfilaria are gone. These medicines are somewhat messy and, not infrequently, cause vomiting or diarrhea, but they are the only ones presently available.

Indoor dogs should be confined to a well-papered area for one hour after each daily treatment, to be sure your dog isn't going to throw up. Once your dog has been freed of both adult worms and microfilaria, he should be put on a *daily* preventive medication throughout the mosquito season, since reinfection can and does occur if such medication is not given.

The preventive drug, *diethylcarbamazine*, is inexpensive and available from your veterinarian in tablet, powder, or liquid form, making its oral administration quite easy and not at all costly. The drug is effective for only one day and has no cumulative effect. If you skip a day and your dog meets an infected mosquito, it is as if you hadn't been giving anything. Dogs living in heavily infected areas, particularly in warmer climes, should be medicated the year-round. In the north, with shorter mosquito seasons, preventive medication should be started just before the season and continued for *two months after* the first killing frost eliminates the mosquitoes. Your veterinarian will blood-test your dog before starting him on diethylcarbamazine to be sure he doesn't already have heartworms. This medication must never be given to an infected dog, as severe and sometimes fatal reactions can take place. If it is not given on a year-round basis, your dog must be blood-tested each year before starting the drug.

In younger dogs, an alternate method of prevention is to give the arsenic injections every six months to kill the young adult worms before they start reproducing. The extra hazards of this therapy in aging dogs has been made clear, and I do not recommend this preventive method for your geriatric dog.

The frequency of blood-testing and length and form of prevention will depend upon where the dog lives and the prevalence of the disease. Your veterinarian will advise you appropriately. The use of screens, insect sprays, and other methods of mosquito control will also help protect your dog from this very serious disease.

7
The Respiratory System

Your dog's lungs have two vitally important functions. They exchange carbon dioxide, one of the body's waste products in the blood, for oxygen from the air breathed in. They also help eliminate excess body heat and water through evaporation and exhalation.

The functional unit of lung tissue, the alveolus, is made up of a very thin membrane with inhaled air on one side and circulating blood on the other side. As carbon dioxide leaves the blood, oxygen enters it from the air side of the membrane. Water and heat can also leave the blood across the alveolar membrane. Anything that interferes with this free two-way passage—the thickening of an inflamed alveolar membrane, excess mucus secretions, infections, tumors, inordinate heat—will reduce the level of oxygen circulating in the blood and cause varying degrees of respiratory difficulty. Disorders in the nose, mouth, and windpipe, as well as outside the respiratory system, can also result in respiratory disease.

Pleural Effusion and Pulmonary Edema

These two conditions are almost always secondary to another primary disease which, in aging dogs, is usually heart failure, lung disease, and tumors in the lungs or chest cavity. Pulmonary edema is an excessive accumulation of fluid in the lung tissues. Pleural effusion is an accumulation of fluid in the very small spaces between the lungs and chest wall. Both conditions greatly reduce lung function, making it increasingly difficult for the dog to breathe.

Heat Stress (Heat Stroke, Sun Stroke)

Both obesity and advancing years reduce a dog's tolerance to extremes of heat. The brachycephalic breeds (those with the pushed-in face) are particularly susceptible, due to their normal respiratory difficulties. It is through respiration that the majority of your dog's excess body heat is eliminated. When you and I get overheated, we breathe rapidly and perspire all over our bodies. Because of their hair coats, dogs are unable significantly to perspire through their skins, although a small amount does occur through the underside of the paws. For all practical purposes, excess body heat must be removed by rapid respiration.

Most dogs, other than the brachycephalics, can withstand exposure to the sun and rather high environmental temperature as long as they are free to move about. It is confinement, restraint, and excitement in hot weather that sets the stage for heat stress. The dog left inside a car in the sun, leashed to a post outside the supermarket, or held in a pen when there are other dogs nearby to excite it, is a prime candidate for this life-threatening emergency.

Symptoms range from panting with a hot *dry* tongue, bright *red* mucous membranes in the mouth, rapid heartbeat, and a hot, dry skin, to a dazed look, inability to stand, unconsciousness, and death. The body temperature may be between 106° and 110°F (41.1°–43.3°C). The chance of death increases in direct proportion to the length of time the body temperature remains that high. This is a true emergency.

Remove the dog from the constraining environment to a cooler place, preferably indoors. Immediately, before anything else is done, telephone your veterinarian. If she is in, and you can get to her clinic *quickly*, go directly there. In the event travel time will be prolonged, she may advise you to start emergency treatment at home, under her telephone direction, and then bring your dog to the clinic. But suppose you cannot reach her by phone—you're camping out miles from a telephone, or she is on vacation and the nearest veterinarian is in another town at a considerable distance. You must take action at once!

The most urgent need is to lower the dog's body temperature. Immerse the *entire* body, except the head, in cold or ice water—a bathtub, stream, river, or lake—anything that has or can hold cold water. Take care to support the dog so he doesn't collapse into the water. Massage the skin all over the body and flex and extend the legs one at a time. This will stimulate the flow of the cooled blood back to the heart, through the internal parts of the body and to the heat sensitive brain. If you have a rectal thermometer handy, check the temperature every seven to ten minutes until it reads 103 °F (39.4 °C). Do *not* cool below that point. The dog should then be removed from the water and the temperature checked with the same frequency for at least three-quarters of an hour, to be sure it doesn't start to go up again. Once the temperature has remained stable for that period of time, take your dog as quickly as possible to a veterinarian *somewhere*. There are important medications which should be given to prevent the many serious complications which can follow heat stress.

There is no excuse for heat stress ever occurring. No one questions your love for your dog, or he wouldn't have survived this long. Just a little logical forethought during hot weather is all that is needed. Don't take him shopping with you if your stores do not allow dogs on the premises. Then you won't have to tie him outside. If you are going for a drive, be sure he will be welcome at every place you intend to stop. If his outdoor exercise area is small, take him indoors before you leave the house for any length of time. Those breeds more prone to heat stress—pug, boxer, English bulldog, Boston terrier, etc.—should have even normal outdoor activity severely curtailed during periods of hot sun and high temperatures. In extremely hot parts of the country they may require air-conditioning. Certainly, free access to frequently changed cool water is a must. As far as I am concerned, any dog who suffers heat stress, and survives, ought to pack up and look for a new owner!

Chronic Bronchitis

A disease seen with increasing frequency in dogs of middle age and older, chronic bronchitis is rarely seen in younger dogs. This disorder should not be confused with viral or bacterial tracheobronchitis, so-called "kennel cough," which *is* very common in the young, although it can occur at any age. The organs involved are the bronchi and bronchioles, those progressively narrowing tubes we all breathe through which connect the trachea, or windpipe, to the lungs. When the normal mucus secretions in those tubes are produced in excess, bronchitis results.

The condition in dogs is very similar to chronic bronchitis in people and is found mainly in the small, but not necessarily toy, breeds. In addition, it is seen with too great a frequency in obese animals. By far the commonest symptom is chronic coughing often followed by gagging and spitting up some of the excess mucus. It can be made worse by any increase in activity, excitement or long periods of *in*activity, as during sleep. Such dogs cough profusely when waking up in the morning and may actually be awakened during the night by a need literally to "clear their throats."

Inasmuch as the cause of chronic bronchitis has yet to be determined, treatment is not always successful and even when it is, recurrences are to be expected. Initial therapy may require hospitalization unless such change in environment causes the dog increased excitement. Antibiotics, confinement and rest, weight reduction, nebulization, and oxygen may be used. Culturing the bronchial secretions is often done to determine which antibiotic will be most effective. When your dog goes home, you must provide a quiet restful atmosphere which will neither excite nor upset him. Among the medications to be given at home may be a cough suppressant. Some coughing is desirable to help move the secretions out of the throat, so do not expect the medicine to stop the coughing completely. To do so could make your dog more ill. In severe cases you may be advised to have a small tank of oxygen at home and will be given full instructions how to use it safely. Remember, oxygen is flammable!

Pneumonia

Dogs of all ages are susceptible to the many causes of this generally serious disease of the lungs. The reason it is included here is that pneumonia often develops in dogs with a prolonged or debilitating illness. The aging dog is more likely to have such illnesses and develop pneumonia as a secondary complication. It can be brought about by many different causative agents—bacteria, viruses, fungus, parasites, allergy, and others. After directing treatment at the primary disorder, therapy for pneumonia is similar to that of chronic bronchitis and may require many weeks of medication.

Tumors

It is sad, but true, that almost all tumors which occur in the lungs or elsewhere within the chest are malignant. This does not, however, mean that all dogs who develop such tumors are irrevocably condemned. Some tumors are quite small and just a single nodule. Diagnosed early, before they have time to metastasize elsewhere, such tumors can quite often be successfully removed. Your family veterinarian will X-ray the chest to determine that the growth is single and shows no sign of having spread. In that case an exploratory operation will be undertaken to confirm this and to be sure that the adjacent lymph nodes are not involved. If these nodes and all other lobes of the lungs, as well as other structures in the chest cavity, appear to be "clean," the entire affected lung lobe will be removed, and the tumor sent to a pathologist for identification. (Positive tumor identification is essential in determining the long-range prognosis.)

Many lung tumors do not show signs of illness until they have spread considerably. In addition, tumors originating elsewhere—kidney, spleen, breast, skin, and bone—are prone to spread rapidly to the lungs. Such affected patients are inoperable, as they would require the removal of more lung than they could live without or else the removal of other vital structures, without which they could not survive. These dogs will be treated as best as possible to alleviate whatever discomfort or disability results from the malignancy. Depending on the type of tumor, such palliative therapy may succeed for many months or perhaps only a few weeks. It is common for many of these dogs to lead relatively normal and, for the dog, happy lives during therapy. However, when the quality of life no longer is normal or happy, the medication becomes ineffective, or pain and suffering begin, treatment should be stopped, and that life humanely brought to an end.

Asthma

To the extent of our present knowledge in veterinary medicine, true bronchial asthma as found in people and certain other animals, does not seem to occur naturally in the dog, although it can be produced experimentally. While some symptoms are often found which may be similar to those of asthma, they have generally have been traced to other primary respiratory diseases.

8
The Urinary System

The digestive and respiratory systems each have, as part of their normal function, the elimination of some of the body's metabolic waste products. But it is the urinary system which has the greatest responsibility in this area and must deal with the major portion of these wastes. Inasmuch as the kidneys slowly start to "age" rather early in life, disorders of the urinary system are very common in older dogs, and kidney disease is a frequent diagnosis. For a long time before the veterinary profession fully understood the cardiovascular and other geriatric diseases of older dogs, kidney disease was considered the primary ailment of aging canines and the most frequent cause of death. It is still one of the commonest geriatric disorders.

Polydipsia–Polyuria

If you happen to observe your veterinarian's notations as she takes down your dog's medical history, you may see the phrase "PD–PU" being written. This shorthand stands for polydipsia, an excessive thirst, and polyuria, an excessive amount of urination. These are not diseases, but rather a pair of symptoms frequently seen together in a wide variety of illnesses. Since they are rather difficult to miss, they will often be among the first abnormal signs you will notice. Among the ailments of aging dogs which are associated with PD–PU are diabetes mellitus, bladder and kidney disease, liver disorders, certain abnormalities of the thyroid, parathyroid and adrenal glands, and the uterine infection known as pyometra. These are discussed in their appropriate sections. Two other ailments which exhibit PD-PU, neither especially common, nor having an increased frequency in older dogs, are diabetes insipidus and psychological thirst.

Cystitis

Inflammation of the urinary bladder, known as cystitis, occurs with some frequency in the aging canine. There may or may not be an infection of the bladder present at the same time. In both males and females, the symptoms include increased frequency of urination, frequent attempts to urinate which produce only small amounts of urine each time, straining or pain during urination, and occasional blood in the urine. In more severe cases, there can also be loss of appetite, vomiting, and listlessness.

There are many possible causes of cystitis such as bladder and urethral stones, bladder tumors, mechanical injury, diabetes mellitus, and others. By far the commonest cause is the prolonged retention of urine in the bladder which reduces the normal acidity of that urine and allows bacteria to multiply rapidly. An all too common reason for urine retention in the well-trained, house-broken dog is inadequate opportunity to get outdoors to eliminate. The older dog, whose kidneys are losing some of their ability to function, as described a bit further on, will drink increasing amounts of water to aid the kidneys with their work load. Hence, more urine will be produced, the bladder will fill faster, and the dog will have to urinate more frequently. By the simple action of getting your dog outdoors more often to allow adequate urination and emptying of the bladder, you can significantly reduce the chances of cystitis developing.

A male dog has one additional and very important source of bladder infection, and that is the prostate gland. The urethra, which comes from the bladder and through which your dog urinates, passes right through the middle of the prostate. Infections of that gland readily enter the urethra and pass back into the bladder. (The prostate gland is fully discussed in chapter 5.)

For diagnosis your veterinarian will do a urinalysis and probably culture the urine. He may also take radiographs of the bladder alone or of the entire urinary tract, from kidneys down to urethra, depending upon the particular causative factors suspected. Following the correction of any causes outside the bladder, your dog will be placed on an appropriate urinary antibiotic for at least three weeks. Bladder infections in your dog take a long time to cure, just as they do in people. It is not uncommon for medication to have to be continued for two or three months.

Urinary acidifiers may also be prescribed, and you may be asked to test the acidity of your dog's urine every day with a special testing paper. This is not as difficult as it may sound. When your dog lifts his leg, or she squats to urinate, you simply hold a strip of the test paper in the stream of urine and then compare it to a color chart on the dispenser it comes in. This will give you the pH number, which measures how acid or alkaline the urine is. Your veterinarian will tell you in which range of numbers the pH test should read and how to adjust the acidifier dosage accordingly. With a little practice you will be able to perform this test quickly and accurately. Frequent laboratory checks of other elements in your dog's urine are sometimes necessary in the treatment of cystitis, as well as other disorders. If your veterinarian asks *you* to collect the specimen at home, you may get far more practice than you had planned on.

Normally, the doctor would collect the urine by passing a catheter through the urethra into the bladder, obtaining a sterile specimen. Even though this is done very carefully, there is always a risk of injuring the delicate membranes which line the urethra and bladder, or possibly introducing bacteria into them. When repeated urine samples are needed, you may be asked to collect them *au naturel*. Thoroughly washed and sterilized (by boiling for thirty minutes) saucers, aluminum pie plates and potato shells, cups, soup ladles, and so on, carefully placed beneath the urine source, have all been successfully used for this task. It may take a lot of patience and ingenuity, but it *can* be done. I'm sure your veterinarian has his own favorite method and will describe it to you in detail.

In the event you simply cannot, or will not, manage to collect your dog's urine, it is very important that you own up to it, tell your doctor, and not try to pass off a substitute specimen. *Don't laugh!* My memory races back to Josephine, of *Every Night, Josephine!* fame. I shared in the pleasure of caring for Josie's health during the eighth year of her long life, when I was an associate doctor in another veterinarian's hospital. I asked Josie's owner, the late Jacqueline Susann, to bring in a morning specimen of her dog's urine, and carefully explained how to collect it. Upon discussing it at home with her husband, Irving Mansfield, they developed a long list of reasons why they couldn't collect Josie's urine. As Miss Susann relates in her book, "we were really doing this to keep the doctors happy. . . ." Hence, Mr. Mansfield arrived the following morning with a full specimen bottle—without a word that it contained his own urine.

Despite the period of treatment often being quite long, most cases of cystitis are eventually cured. The one exception is cystitis caused by a bladder tumor. If diagnosed while it is still small, the tumor and a substantial portion of the surrounding bladder can be removed and still leave enough bladder to function adequately. It is often the case, however, that these tumors cause no noticeable signs when they are small, and by the time abnormal symptoms are apparent, they are too large to be removed without taking out the entire bladder. Also by that time, they probably will have spread to other organs, since a high percentage of such tumors are malignant. Chemotherapy and immunotherapy can be given to control the tumor for short periods and alleviate the symptoms for a while.

Incontinence

An infrequent difficulty in older female dogs, who have had an ovariohysterectomy done, is to lose some or all of their voluntary control of the act of urinating. Urine will dribble out while they are lying down and sometimes even while they are walking; the dog most often is totally unaware of it. The exact cause is as yet undetermined and, even though it responds to estrogen therapy, lack of estrogens has not been proven to be the cause. The administration of oral estrogen in very low doses about once a week or by injection monthly or bimonthly, depending on response, will almost always bring bladder control back to normal. This therapy will have to continue for the rest of your dog's life. As you well know, estrogens can cause several blood abnormalities and, in women, cause predisposition to certain types of cancer. Your veterinarian will want to blood-test your dog at regular intervals to preclude the possibility of any such undesirable effects.

In the aging male dog, incontinence is only occasionally found secondary to cystitis, prostatitis, intervertebral disc disease, and other conditions discussed elsewhere. It may also be found in cases of urethral or bladder stones, which dogs of both sexes and *all* ages sometimes develop.

Kidney Disorders

The paired kidneys of the dog, like those of almost all animals, perform several tasks. The two primary and most important ones are the conservation of the body's water content and vital chemicals; and the elimination from the body of harmful chemicals and the waste products which result from metabolism, especially of protein. These functions are accomplished by filtering the blood through the approximately four hundred thousand functional units, called nephrons, which make up *each* kidney. The end product of this filtration process is urine which, in your normal healthy dog, is produced at the average rate of fifteen milliliters or one-half fluid ounce per day for each pound of body weight.

The kidneys have an enormous reserve capacity, much like the liver, but unlike that organ, they have relatively little ability to regenerate, once damaged. Instead, they heal by forming nonfunctional scar tissue. There is so much reserve, that a dog can function quite normally with only one healthy kidney, as when a tumor in the other one requires its removal. In fact, as little as one-third of the kidneys' nephrons are all that are needed to maintain normal function. The other two-thirds can be severely damaged and nonfunctional. The viable part compensates quite adequately for the injured part. Because of this, progressive chronic kidney disease can exist for a long time without any observable symptoms. Early detection based only on history and physical examination can be very difficult, but the routine preventive laboratory tests performed in an annual geriatric exam may identify such early changes.

KIDNEY DISEASE VS. KIDNEY FAILURE

The term kidney disease is used to refer to all abnormalities, involving any number of nephrons, of one or both kidneys, regardless of the specific cause. Kidney failure occurs when seventy-five percent, or more, of the nephrons of *both* kidneys have been completely damaged, the remaining portion can no longer compensate, and therefore the kidneys can no longer sustain life. Once renal failure occurs, regardless of the actual cause, the harmful chemicals and waste products cannot be eliminated from the body, and an autointoxication or self-poisoning—uremia—predictably takes place.

Many of the symptoms of uremia can be found in diseases of other organs and are rarely pathognomonic for kidney disease or failure. Alterations in respiration and heart function, dehydration, anemia, ulcers in the mouth, a sweetish odor to the breath, pain over the kidneys, demineralization of bone, vomiting, diarrhea, polydipsia–polyuria, depression, and, occasionally, convulsions have all been reported to occur in uremic dogs. All or none of these may be present in any given canine. Severe changes in the balance of sodium, potassium, and body fluids, plus the accumulation of metabolic waste products, appear to be the causes of death in renal failure.

The dog with kidney failure almost always will require in-hospital treatment because of the necessary intensive therapy, frequent examination, and testing that must be done. Diagnostic procedures, in addition to a complete history and physical exam, will include at least some of the following: a urinalysis and culture, blood chemistry tests such as urea nitrogen or creatinine concentrations, kidney function tests, contrast and noncontrast X-ray studies, or a kidney biopsy. In some of the more difficult to diagnose cases, all of these and others may be necessary.

A dog who recovers from kidney disease has nevertheless lost some of his functional nephrons. The remaining nephrons undergo compensation to perform the extra work. One way of eliminating more waste product is to allow more water to pass through the kidneys, thus "washing out" the wastes with it. For this reason the dog with renal disease makes much more urine—polyuria. In order to make up for this excess loss of body fluid, the dog drinks more water—polydipsia—and we have the PD-PU pattern so often observed in most kinds of kidney disease. The increased water intake may result in nocturia—urination during the night, either asleep or awake. By not providing sufficient drinking water, in order to "cut down on so much urinating," you can cause decompensation and quickly precipitate an acute life-threatening episode of kidney failure. A dog with compensated kidney disease must not be deprived of water!

CAUSES OF KIDNEY DISEASE

The causes of kidney disease can be divided into three groups, based on general location of the initiating problem, namely prerenal, postrenal, and primary renal disease.

In postrenal disease, the disorder arises in that part of the urinary tract beyond the kidneys—the ureters, which connect the kidneys to the bladder, the bladder itself, or the urethra. Partial or complete obstruction, by stones or tumors, prevents elimination of the urine that the kidneys are producing. Prolonged obstruction rapidly damages otherwise normal kidneys. While such problems can occur at any age, they are not seen very frequently in aged dogs.

Prerenal disorders occur outside the urinary tract and before the blood reaches the kidneys to be filtered. In the aged dog, the main cause is a poorly functioning heart. Kidney function depends, among other things, on an adequate rate of blood flowing through the nephrons. Many forms of heart disease result in lowered blood pressure, which can cause a proportionate decrease in the filtration rate of the otherwise normal kidneys. Should the pressure fall below a certain critical level, all filtration ceases, little if any urine is produced, and renal failure and uremia ensue.

Primary renal disease occurs with the kidney proper, being the result of infections, chemical or other poisons, or tumors. Recently, it has been suggested that defects in a dog's immune mechanisms can also cause primary renal disease. A sudden episode of renal failure, from whatever cause, holds out a more favorable prognosis for recovery than chronic kidney failure which is usually progressive and irreversible, therefore permitting a far less favorable prognosis.

Both primary and secondary causes of kidney disease exist. Bacterial infection from within or outside the urinary tract occurs frequently, and viral infection is rarely involved. Many chemicals have a specific toxic effect on the kidneys, among them being lead, arsenic, carbon tetrachloride (cleaning fluid), and ethylene glycol (antifreeze). Under certain circumstances, some antibiotics can also poison the kidneys. Whenever your veterinarian prescribes these antibiotics, he will give you very specific instructions on their use. Many diseases which affect all or large parts of the body (systemic) can produce kidney disease. Among these are diabetes mellitus, heart disease, pyometra, leptospirosis, and some immune mechanism diseases like systemic lupus erythematosis.

Because renal disease can result from such a wide variety of causes arising in so many different parts of the body, there is really very little you can specifically do to prevent it other than keeping your dog from contact with the known kidney-poisonous chemicals. Infections are also difficult to prevent other than insuring ample amounts of drinking water and immediately investigating any significant reduction of water intake or urine output. Of course, the annual geriatric exam may detect renal disease in its early stages when therapy is most effective.

CHRONIC INTERSTITIAL NEPHRITIS OR END STAGE KIDNEY DISEASE

Repeated bouts of kidney disease in the older dog cause progressive deterioration of renal function and result in a disease complex formerly called chronic interstitial nephritis but now more descriptively referred to as end stage kidney disease. It is considerably more common in males than in females for reasons unknown. The compensated status of diseased kidneys is a precarious one at best. *Any* form of stress can upset the balance, cause decompensation, and precipitate a renal crisis. Undue excitement, extremes of weather, inadequate water, urine retention, and sudden increases in the amount of dietary protein are some of the more frequent causes. In addition to depression, weakness, vomiting, and diarrhea, there may be a *reduction* in the volume of urine being produced.

Many of the precipitating causes of renal failure crises are reversible for varying periods and should be managed as described in the next paragraph. Some, however, will have little potential for such reversibility, and to undertake the necessary effort and expense such treatment would incur might not be warranted. Your veterinarian will discuss with you, in all candor, the possible potential for a successful outcome and recommend therapy, no therapy, or euthanasia, as the case seems to indicate in his judgment. With his help, you must make the choice.

There is currently no treatment that will stop or reverse the progress of end stage kidney disease. Yet your veterinarian, with your help, can often establish a regimen of medication, diet, and activity which will minimize the work load of the functioning nephrons, prolonging their ability to maintain a reasonably comfortable life for months and sometimes years.

The initial treatment of a renal crisis will be done in the veterinary hospital, but once a balanced and stable metabolic status is reestablished, you will be able to take your dog home. Be certain to get complete and detailed instructions for home care. I recommend you write them down in order to avoid any misunderstanding or misinterpretation. There is no margin for error in the treatment of chronic renal failure.

The important aspects of successfully maintaining your dog can be characterized as follows:

- Provide as little work as possible for the remaining functional nephrons.
- Prevent dehydration from loss of body fluids.
- Replace the sodium and other salts lost in the urine.
- Supplement the diet with certain vitamins also lost in the urine.
- Avoid stress.

The bulk of the kidneys' work results from processing the end products of protein metabolism whereas carbohydrate and fat metabolism produces little work for them. Low protein diets are, therefore, used regularly in treating renal failure. Readily digestible protein of high biological value should be fed in amounts just adequate to supply the necessary amino acids. Sufficient energy producing calories from carbohydrates and fats must also be provided, so that proteins are not broken down for energy. Such diets are commercially available either from, or on the prescription of, your veterinarian and can be had in canned, semimoist or dry form. Alas, they are not highly palatable, and your aged dog, grown accustomed to a particular diet over the years, may not take kindly to these prescription foods. Should this be a problem, a homemade special diet can be used, with the approval, and under the supervision, of your veterinarian. You must, however, resist the strong temptation, which often arises, to alter the established recipe "just a little bit." That "little bit" could be enough to trigger a uremic crisis. Eggs, lean meats, cottage cheese, and chicken are good sources of high biological value protein. Good carbohydrates and fats include spaghetti and noodles, rice, cake, cream cheese, ice cream, vegetable oil, and bread. Your veterinarian will help you select the right amounts of each food to be included in the diet *every* day; these should not be changed except at his instruction. As time goes on and additional nephrons are damaged, it may be necessary to reduce the protein content further.

Because failing kidneys make large quantities of urine in their efforts to compensate, proportionate amounts of water are lost from the body. In order to prevent dehydration, your dog must have *continuous* free access to fresh drinking water, unless she is vomiting. The outdoor dog should have it available outside or be able to get into the house by herself to get it there—she cannot wait for someone to open the door for her. If you must be out all day or for the evening, put out several large water dishes to be sure there will be enough until your return. I do not recommend teaching your dog to drink from the toilet bowl, no matter how clean you may think that water source is; and if you leave a faucet running slowly, you may come home to find a flood. In hot weather, you can expect her to drink more, just as a healthy dog would.

Sodium, bicarbonate, chloride, and other chemicals are also lost in the increased urination. You will be advised how much table salt or other additives *your* dog will need daily. It will vary from dog to dog but can be mixed right in with the special diet.

Supplementation of the water soluble vitamins, such as the B-vitamins and ascorbic acid, will also be recommended.

Stress of any kind must be avoided if at all possible. Don't change the environment, even to the point of not rearranging furniture or redecorating. Moving to a new home has been known to cause a renal crisis. Any illness, particularly those which are infectious, or cause fever or loss of appetite, can adversely affect a compensated renal state. How to avoid stress will vary with your individual sitution and life-style, but your family veterinarian will advise you to the best of his ability on ways to accomplish this goal.

As the number of functional nephrons diminishes, despite the above maintenance regimen, it may become necessary, in order to save your dog's life, to assist the kidneys. There are three basic methods of doing this. The intravenous injection of a drug which stimulates the excretion of water and metabolic wastes is called osmotic diuresis and is usually the first technique used. If this fails to do the job, or if complete renal shutdown occurs and *no* urine is being produced, kidney function must be provided artificially. Peritoneal dialysis is a technique which causes the transfer of water and wastes out of the body's tissues and into the abdominal cavity from where it is physically removed. It is slower than osmotic diuresis and often has to be repeated several times a day for the first few days. Under local anesthesia along the abdominal wall, a tube is inserted into the abdomen, and a special dialyzing fluid is directed into the abdomen where it is left for about an hour. The waste products pass from the tissues into the dialyzing fluid which is then slowly removed through the same tube. Once stabilized, and when the kidneys again are able to compensate, the tube is removed. In effect, peritoneal dialysis is a lower cost substitute for the artificial kidney machines used in human medicine. Due to the economics involved, as well as technical problems relating to their use in dogs, such machines are not yet practical for routine use in canine kidney patients.

When all else fails, it is theoretically possible to replace at least one of the nonfunctioning kidneys by transplantation of a healthy one from a suitable donor dog. All the techniques and technology used in performing a kidney transplant in humans were researched, developed, and perfected first, in dogs. Unfortunately, the same problem of the body rejecting the new kidney, which occurs in people, is also found in the canine patient. In fact, it appears that the dog has an even more involved system of transplant rejection than does the human. Even with immunosuppressive drugs and radiation therapy, survival time before rejection can be measured in only days or weeks. A lot more must be learned about organ compatibility, rejection mechanisms, and immunosuppression, before a kidney transplant can become a practical and life saving reality for the dog in kidney failure.

KIDNEY TUMORS

Tumors can develop in the kidneys, as in any other organ of the body, and may arise independently in the tissues of either one or both kidneys. Since virtually all the body's blood supply eventually flows through the kidneys, tumor cells are readily carried there from primary tumors often at great distances elsewhere in the body.

Primary renal tumors may be benign, cause little if any noticeable disease, and are uncommon. Malignant primary tumors are more frequently seen, and the chance of occurrence increases with advancing age. Many types do occur, but carcinoma is the commonest primary malignancy of the kidneys. It spreads readily, especially to the liver, lungs, and the other kidney. In the early stages, symptoms are vague or nonexistent except for occasional blood in the urine of an otherwise healthy-appearing dog. As more of the kidney is destroyed, PD–PU, vomiting, weight loss, and all the other symptoms of chronic kidney disease may be observed.

If the tumor is in only one kidney, has not metastasized elsewhere, and the other kidney is healthy enough to function normally, the diseased kidney and its ureter can be surgically removed with good results. On the other hand, if both kidneys are cancerous, the tumor has spread, or the opposite kidney is itself failing, surgery cannot be considered, and the prognosis is indeed grave. Radiation therapy, chemotherapy, or both can be helpful in prolonging life. See the further discussions in chapter 14.

9
Disorders of Metabolism

Your dog's body is a highly developed and very complex chemical "factory," which is continually building up (anabolism) and tearing down (catabolism) his own living tissue, producing energy as well as waste products from the food and water he ingests and the oxygen he breathes. The sum total of all these reactions is called metabolism, and they are controlled principally by hormones produced in many different parts of the body. These hormones regulate the *rate* at which the reactions occur. Any increase or decrease in the production of a given hormone alters metabolism by causing a proportional change in the specific reactions it regulates.

Some of the commoner hormones you may know and their sources are listed here. Keep in mind, however, that there are many, many more.

Hormone	*Produced By*
Insulin	Pancreas
Corticosteroid	Adrenal gland
Thyroxin	Thyroid gland
Growth hormone	Pituitary gland
Epinephrine (adrenalin)	Adrenal gland
Estrogen	Ovary
Testosterone	Testicle

Although diseases of the ovaries and testicles often cause disorders of metabolism, they are discussed in chapter 5.

Diabetes mellitus

So-called sugar or glucose diabetes, properly known as diabetes mellitus, is probably the most common metabolic disorder of dogs and is seen most often during the middle and late years of life. Both sexes are susceptible, but there is an almost five-fold greater frequency in females. This higher incidence prevails whether or not the bitch has had an ovariohysterectomy. Poodles, cocker spaniels, and dachshunds develop diabetes with a much higher frequency, although it has been observed in virtually every breed. Yet, for unknown reasons, the boxer dog is notably absent from that list. There is no proof of any hereditary basis, but circumstantial evidence points to the likelihood of a limited familial predisposition. One all too common denominator and major predisposing factor found in large numbers of diabetic dogs is *obesity*.

Diabetes mellitus cannot be cured but can be effectively controlled if diagnosed and treated early. Delay in starting therapy, or haphazard administration of that therapy, will most assuredly result in a life-threatening crisis.

The causes of diabetes are complex, often multiple, and oddly enough, not well understood even today. Recent work has shown it to be more than just an insufficient production of insulin by the pancreas. Regardless, whatever the causes may be, the net result is less insulin than the body requires for its metabolic processes. This results in a build-up of glucose in the bloodstream—hyperglycemia—and eventually it is eliminated in the urine. This is usually accompanied by increased drinking and urination, as well as increased food intake which is attended by a *loss* in weight. In the obese dog, this weight loss may not be apparent until well on in the course of the disease. Any of these signs which persist for more than two days without an *obvious* cause should get you on the phone to your family veterinarian for advice and most likely to arrange for an examination.

In addition to a complete physical exam, blood and urine tests for glucose, other chemicals, and certain enzymes will be done on your dog. This will confirm the diagnosis of diabetes and rule out, or rule in, similar-appearing ailments such as primary kidney disease and disorders of the adrenal or pituitary glands. Liver function tests, as well as X rays of that organ, will be done to determine the extent of its enlargement and malfunction; a common finding in diabetes.

These diagnostic procedures may or may not require your dog to be hospitalized, but, once confirmed, the initial diabetes control and stabilization must be done in the hospital. Repeated blood and urine testing throughout the two to four days it will take, adjusting the dose of insulin and amount of food, and watching for dangerous side reactions cannot safely be done on an out-patient basis.

Once stabilized, your dog will be sent home for continuing daily treatment for the rest of her life. *You* are the key to maintaining that life for as long as possible, and it is a responsibility not to be taken lightly. While it rarely will demand any significant alteration in your life-style, you or someone must be available every day to test the urine, administer the correct dose of insulin by injection, and effectively control diet and exercise—holidays, vacations, your illness, or anything else, notwithstanding. Like any new thing you must get used to, with patience and practice you'll find it fairly simple to do all the things needed to give your dog those additional years of what can be an essentially normal and happy life. Oral medications to lower blood sugar, which can be used in most people, have not only failed in dogs, but at least one type of such medicine is toxic to the canine liver and therefore dangerous. It is hoped that in time a safe and effective oral drug will be developed. Until then insulin must be administered in an injectable form.

Your veterinarian will teach you how to give the injection subcutaneously (under the skin, not in the muscle) as well as recommend ways of catching your dog in the act of urination. You will either be supplied with or be given a prescription for insulin, insulin syringes, and needles depending on your local drug abuse control laws. Insulin must be kept refrigerated at all times and the bottle shaken very well *immediately* before use. If disposable syringes are prescribed, they are intended for one use only and should be destroyed in a manner your doctor will explain to you.

In the event glass syringes are prescribed, they must be washed and sterilized after *each* use as per your doctor's instructions. You will also be told what kind of urine testing paper to buy in the pharmacy and how to use it.

The specific details of the course of treatment for diabetes must be individually determined for *your* dog—there is no one set of procedures for all diabetics. Your veterinarian will probably give you written instructions which should be followed exactly. It will include how and when to test the urine; how to adjust the insulin dose, which can vary from day to day; when to give the insulin; and when to feed your dog in relation to the time of injection. A sample routine might be as follows:

1. Test your dog's urine first thing in the morning.
2. Give the adjusted insulin dose by subcutaneous injection.
3. Feed one-half of the total daily food.
4. In the evening, feed the other half of the food.

Some dogs may require insulin twice a day in divided doses or need more frequent feedings. It is safer for a dog to have a slightly elevated blood sugar than to have too low a level. Therefore, the goal in treating a diabetic is, *not* to eliminate all the glucose from the urine, but rather to keep the daily urine test slightly positive.

A vital part of the therapy is the diet, which must remain constant from day to day, both in amount and type of food, so the caloric intake does not change. You must take precautions that children—yours or the neighbors—and well-meaning visitors don't feed anything to a diabetic dog. Any such change will radically alter the body's insulin needs, so no snacks or stealing from the table. Unless your dog requires special diets because of concurrent kidney, heart, or other disease, she should be fed a good quality high protein, low carbohydrate commercial dog food. In the presence of obesity, your veterinarian will help you to determine the amount of food which will both reduce the dog and balance the insulin.

It is important that your dog finish all the food provided. Too little food will cause the same effect as if too much insulin had been given, namely, abnormally low blood glucose or hypoglycemia. Symptoms resemble a state of drunkenness and include weakness, dizziness, staggering, uncoordinated gait, and, in severe cases, convulsions or coma. At the earliest sign of *any* of these, immediately give Karo Syrup® by mouth, one tablespoonful for each five pounds of dog. If she cannot swallow or is convulsing or in a coma, smear the syrup on her gums and inside the cheeks. The sugar in the syrup will be rapidly absorbed from those tissues without the need to swallow it. If the dog is not significantly improved within thirty minutes or the symptoms get worse, call your veterinarian regardless of the time of day or night.

Exercise must be controlled and kept fairly constant from day to day. The easiest way to do this is to keep your dog on a leash and walk or jog for a set length of time as advised by your doctor. If your dog is accustomed to roaming the neighborhood, it will be necessary to stop this unsupervised outdoor activity. Any sudden spurt of physical movement, like chasing another dog, will quickly burn up large amounts of energy and glucose. In what can be only a matter of minutes in a critically stabilized dog, hypoglycemia is likely to occur along with all its potentially hazardous consequences.

Special problems exist for the unspayed diabetic female. Every time she goes through her heat cycle, control of the diabetic condition becomes very difficult and precarious as the delicate insulin-diet balance is completely upset. This can quickly lead to another severe complication called ketoacidosis, an emergency situation which is often fatal. It is therefore important for intact diabetic bitches to have an ovariohysterectomy performed as soon as possible after their initial stabilization.

Cataracts occur with some frequency in canines who become diabetic. They develop rapidly and can cause blindness even after the diabetes has been controlled. If only one eye becomes cataractous, it is best left alone. However, if both eyes are involved, surgical removal of the cataracts *might* be considered. (See discussions in chapter 10.)

In view of the fact that the causes of diabetes mellitus are not yet clearly understood, there is little one can do to prevent it, but for one glaring exception. There is no question that obesity is somehow related to diabetes in countless cases. Keep your dog's diet reasonable and her waistline trim, and she will have a better chance of never developing this dangerous but controllable disease.

You may hear of another type of diabetes which has nothing to do with sugar or insulin. It is called diabetes insipidus and is the result of an abnormality in the hypothalamus, located just below the brain. Polydipsia and polyuria are the hallmarks of this disorder which is also treated by regular injections, but not of insulin. This diabetes is not particularly common and has no special predilection for older dogs.

Hyperinsulinism

Just as too little insulin causes illness, an excess of this hormone also produces serious disability. In the aging dog, the primary cause is a tumor of the insulin-secreting cells of the pancreas, referred to as an insuloma. The boxer breed, which has a special predilection for many types of tumors, is also more frequently represented among insuloma cases.

The presence of increased insulin causes hypoglycemia and the same symptoms as overdosing or underfeeding a diabetic dog—muscle weakness especially in the hind legs, dizziness, uncoordination, and seizures. In addition, muscle twitching, violent running or barking, yelping as if in pain, and hysteria may occur. These symptoms take place on and off, in the early stages, with intervals of days or weeks but become more frequent and sometimes continuous as the disease progresses. Prolonged or untreated, irreversible brain damage will result.

During its early development it is very difficult to diagnose an insuloma, yet this is when a diagnosis must be made if any therapy is to have a chance at succeeding. Your keen observation of your dog for any suggestive abnormalities is a prerequisite. He walks, runs, and plays as always but then unexpectedly seems to lose interest and be tired. Or he stops suddenly and stands there with his back muscles twitching. His hind legs seem unable to hold him up, and the hind quarters start swaying and collapsing. He lies down for a short time, but soon he is suddenly himself again. You think, "I guess he's just getting old and running out of steam." That could be true, but he may actually be running out of glucose—hypoglycemia—because of an insuloma. Get your dog examined as soon as you can. In the meantime, write down all of those somewhat vague signs which have been occurring on and off, so you can give your veterinarian an accurate history.

Once he suspects the possibility of the existence of an insuloma, your veterinarian will likely conduct a fasting blood sugar test in addition to others. Since this requires your dog to go without food for at least twelve and sometimes twenty-four hours, it is best done in the hospital and may require several days of repeated testing to obtain conclusive information. A single low, normal, or high fasting blood glucose means nothing. If confirmatory of an insuloma, your doctor will then do a test to assay the actual level of insulin in your dog. This somewhat sophisticated test has only recently become available to the veterinary profession on a practical level. With it we can just about pinpoint the existence of an insuloma.

On the surface it would appear that a cure is simple—just remove the tumor. That is often easier said than done. In the canine, the majority of insulomas are malignant and spread rapidly to neighboring lymph nodes and the liver. Removal of the tumor not infrequently will cause a postoperative inflammation of the pancreas—acute pancreatitis—which itself can be life threatening. Since these tumors generally occur at an advanced age, the surgical risk is increased, due to other concurrent disease. Medical therapy is no more successful, as it can only relieve the symptoms, but cannot cure. What then?

Your veterinarian will explain and discuss with you all the factors involved, and together you will decide upon a course. In general, an exploratory operation is attempted if the surgical risk is within reason. If the tumor is readily removable and has not spread, it will be taken out. In the event the surgeon finds the tumor inoperable, or that it has indeed metastatised to other organs, he will take a small bit of it for biopsy and close your dog back up. In either case, the tumor tissue will be sent to a pathologist to determine whether or not it is malignant—not all insulomas are.

Following successful surgery, there is a small, but real, chance of recurrence if the tissue is malignant. Should surgery fail or not be attempted at all, temporary medical therapy should be given to control the abnormal symptoms. The very few drugs that can be used are still experimental in dogs and are likely to lose their effectiveness as the dog builds up a tolerance to them. Life expectancy may be a matter of only a few months. Both an older drug, now being tried in a new way, and a new anticancer drug are presently being researched and hold out considerable promise for the successful medical control, and perhaps cure, of insuloma in the future.

Canine Cushing Syndrome

In 1932, a physician by the name of Harvey Cushing described a condition in people called hyperadrenocorticism, an excessive production of certain corticosteroid secretions of the outer layer of the paired adrenal glands. It quickly became known by the doctor's name, and since the condition in dogs is almost, but not quite, identical to that in humans, we call it Cushing or Cushing-like syndrome. It is caused by excessive, but not tumorous, growth of both glands or, less frequently, by an actual tumor of one or both glands. A tumor in the pituitary gland can also stimulate excess adrenal growth.

In the middle to advanced stages of this disease, the symptoms are "classical." One sees a symmetrical thinning, and then total loss, of hair on both sides of the body, especially on the abdomen and flanks; a thinning of the skin; and the development of a large sagging abdomen. The dog is not obese, only the belly is big. Increased appetite, darkening of the skin and hair color, lethargy, and a lowered resistance to infection may also be present. In the male, the testicles generally shrink in size, and in the female, the clitoris may enlarge and protrude from the vulva. Increased thirst and urination, already described in several other diseases, are usually the only *early* symptoms in canine Cushing syndrome.

Those cases caused by a pituitary gland tumor will often also exhibit aimless wandering about the house, apparent loss of intelligence, pressing of the head against a stationary object such as a wall, and other signs of brain disorder. This is due to the close proximity of the pituitary gland to the brain, sitting as it does directly beneath that organ.

In rare cases, the prolonged administration of corticosteroid medications for the treatment of other conditions can cause some of the symptoms of canine Cushing syndrome. These usually disappear when the medication is stopped.

A number of blood and urine tests are available to distinguish the early polydipsia and polyuria in canine Cushing syndrome from that of kidney, liver, thyroid, and other organ diseases which share the PD–PU symptoms. Definitive diagnosis is usually made by measuring the amount of corticosteroid hormones in the blood and another type of steroid in the urine. Despite the fact that all I have said so far seems to make it sound like an easy thing correctly to diagnose canine Cushing syndrome, the long-range assessment and therapy of positive cases is most difficult.

For the past seven or eight years, a drug known as O,p'-DDD has been used experimentally, but very successfully, to treat and control this disease. The drug selectively destroys certain of the outer layers of the adrenal glands thus reducing their corticosteroid production. Although initial therapy is normally done in the hospital, you, as a cooperative and diligent owner, may be able to do this for your dog at home. Discuss this possibility with your veterinarian, as your dog may be one of those who does better in his own environment. Happily, O,p'-DDD can be given by mouth, but the dose must be calculated based on an accurate weight of your dog and administered each day. You will also have to measure the amount of water he drinks each day and keep a record of it for your doctor who will examine and blood test your dog after five or six days and again when most of the symptoms have subsided. The initial daily treatment for most dogs will take from a week to a week and a half.

When all tests show the hyperadrenocorticism to be under control, medication will be reduced to once a week for the rest of your dog's life. Most symptoms will be gone, and hair will begin to regrow in about eight weeks. During the first six months, he should be examined and blood tested at two-month intervals, and your records of water consumption be given to your doctor for evaluation. From then on, your dog ought to be examined once every six months indefinitely.

In rare cases, O,p'-DDD may destroy more of the adrenal gland than is desired, producing an insufficiency of secretion instead of an excess. Symptoms resemble those of acute kidney and gastrointestinal illness, but in the Cushing dog, you should assume that to be due to an overdose of medication until your doctor proves otherwise. Vomiting, diarrhea, weakness, dehydration, and depression can quickly lead to coma and death, so contact your veterinarian immediately. Just on the remote chance that it might not be possible, ask your doctor in advance to give you a small emergency supply of an appropriate corticosteroid drug to have on hand, along with instructions for use, should overdose symptoms occur.

Even with the availability of O,p'-DDD, those cases involving an adrenal gland tumor should have the affected gland surgically removed. Such operations are generally successful, offering a good prognosis after the initially difficult to control period immediately following surgery. A less optimistic prognosis has to be given when both adrenal glands must be removed. This will make your dog a permanent adrenal-secretion-insufficient patient who must have continuous replacement of the missing secretions. This is accomplished at first by injections and then by implants under the skin every three to six months. Removal of the adrenal glands is quite difficult, as is the early postoperative management. These factors, as well as the expenses involved, should be thoroughly discussed with your veterinarian. If surgery is decided against, O,p'-DDD can be tried, but its effectiveness in adrenal tumor patients has not yet been fully assessed.

For those quite rare Cushing cases caused by a pituitary gland tumor, only surgery will help. Such a procedure is almost like brain surgery and is very dangerous. I do not recommend it be done except in extenuating circumstances—a valuable and still breeding stud dog or personal reasons of emotion which demand everything possible be tried regardless of risk. Unless your family veterinarian is thoroughly experienced in this extremely difficult operation, he will refer you to a veterinary surgeon or neurosurgeon certified by the American College of Veterinary Surgeons. Postoperative care also includes lifelong replacement of certain of the pituitary hormones. As of now, it is best, in my opinion, to keep dogs with such tumors comfortable for as long as is possible and then allow a peaceful death, or, if that is not possible, a painless euthanasia.

Thyroid Tumors

Although far from a common disorder, tumors of the paired thyroid glands do occur more frequently in the canine age group we are concerned with. There are two types of tumors seen. The functional thyroid tumor is rather small, rarely more than one to two inches, benign, and secretes excessive amounts of thyroid hormone. The resulting condition, called functional hyperthyroidism, manifests itself either quite suddenly or very slowly and almost imperceptibly over a long time. The most frequent signs are increased urination, weakness, weight loss in spite of an increased appetite, increased sensitivity to heat, and occasionally nervousness. Complete surgical removal of the tumor brings about a return to normal. Should it be necessary to remove both glands, replacement thyroid hormones must be given indefinitely.

The nonfunctional thyroid tumor does not secrete excess hormone yet is far more dangerous, as most of these are malignant. Once again the boxer breed has a statistically greater incidence of these tumors than all other breeds. These malignant tumors are generally many times larger than the hormone secreting ones and tend to occur in only one gland at a time, although both glands can be tremendously enlarged. Most patients are not seen in the early stages when surgery is best done. When the tumor is as big or bigger than a man's fist, surgery is difficult, dangerous, and not likely to be entirely successful. By this time, it has probably metastasized to other organs, particularly the lungs. Under these circumstances, one can expect an extension of life of only three to eighteen months.

10
The Eyes

It may come as a surprise to you that your dog is quite myopic (near-sighted). This is true of virtually all dogs, but the pushed-in faced (brachycephalic) breeds are more near-sighted than their longer faced cousins. Dogs also have a substantial amount of astigmatism. And although you may be certain she can clearly tell the difference between red, green, and yellow, your dog is actually color blind, seeing different colors as varying shades and intensities of gray. For these reasons, among others, her visual acuity is not very good compared to that of humans, and her vision depends more upon shape, motion, and relative brightness. Yet her depth perception is relatively good. Do you remember those younger days when she could leap up and unfailingly grasp a thrown ball, stick, or morsel of food in mid-air? The normal and abnormal changes related to aging can further reduce visual acuity to varying degrees.

Blindness

The majority of eye problems unique to, or found primarily in, older dogs lead to variable degrees of vision loss or total blindness. For the dog, however, blindness rarely ever becomes the severe handicap as it so often is in people. In the first place, your dog doesn't have to read the *New York Times*, watch the "Late Show," or play golf. Because of his naturally greater senses of hearing and smell, upon which he depended more than on his sight even when his eyes were normal, he can now trust them to guide him about with relative ease.

There are very few extra things you have to do to help him. Perhaps the most critical is that you not move or rearrange furniture or other physical objects that he has become used to when vision was still present. He will remember their location and be able slowly to navigate around them. Most blind dogs do *not* bump into things unless they are forced to move too quickly. You should always speak to your blind dog when you are approaching so as not to startle him. Children especially should be taught not to touch him suddenly without first speaking. Such sudden contact could be misinterpreted as a threat and cause your dog to snap or bite.

A dog who has lost part or all of its sight can still lead a very happy and normal life. I really get shook up by a dog owner who requests euthanasia of such a dog because "he's getting in the way." Euthanasia should *never* be considered solely on the basis of blindness!

Fredi, a delightful miniature poodle, became totally and inoperably blind when she was ten. Unlike most geriatric dogs, she was really "showing her age" because of several earlier serious illnesses. Yet she was alert and playful during her waking hours. She enjoyed life and was able to locate food and water dishes with pinpoint accuracy and most everything else in the house without stumbling into anything. About two years after the onset of blindness, it became necessary for Fredi's owner to move to a nearby suburb. Panic set in at the thought of Fredi trying to move about in totally new surroundings. Even I was somewhat apprehensive about the outcome. Once again, love of dog, personal commitment, and resolve brought joy and happiness for all concerned out of a situation fraught with peril for Fredi.

This resourceful client each day before and after work literally walked Fredi through one room at a time. First she took her around the periphery of each room to learn where the doorways were and then, one by one, to each piece of furniture, letting the dog smell and paw at each. In a little more than a month of this, Fredi was able to maneuver very slowly throughout the apartment with only occasional mishaps. Reinforcement of this introduction technique was continued in problem areas; and three months after moving in, one would swear Fredi had lived in that new apartment all of her life. She even learned safely to enjoy a small back yard. It was as if she never left the old place! At almost fourteen years of age she was still going strong!

Nuclear Sclerosis and Cataracts

There have been many occasions when an obviously upset client has brought his dog in for examination because he just noticed her eyes were becoming bluish and was afraid the dog was "going blind" from cataracts. It always pleases me to be able to explain, in most cases, that the dog neither has cataracts nor is going blind. Such dogs have nuclear sclerosis, which is quite different from cataracts in both development and potential problems. The structural fibers which make up the lens of each eye are continually growing and undergoing changes throughout life. The newly produced fibers tend to push the older ones toward the thicker central portion of the lens. This increases the central density, making the lens reflect light somewhat differently but *not* altering its ability to transmit light. The result is a slightly bluish haze one sees when the light catches the eye just right. Increasing age also brings with it some degree of lens dehydration, adding further to the central density. This is, not cataract formation, but rather nuclear sclerosis of the lens, a *normal* aging process.

Most dogs normally have poor central visual acuity, seeing mainly through the noncentral portions of the lens. Inasmuch as nuclear sclerosis develops centrally but remains translucent, there is very little interference with vision. In extreme age, it is possible for these changes to progress toward the periphery, but they rarely ever involve the total lens, and some sight will still remain. No type of treatment is necessary.

Cataracts are an entirely different story. By definition, they are "opacities of the crystalline lens of the eye" which do not transmit light and may be partial or complete, congenital or developmental. They occur at any age and are divided into many classifications and subdivisions. We will concern ourselves here only with the cataract of growing old, the so-called senile cataract. Let me hasten to say that this term classifies the abnormal lens and in no way implies that the dog is senile in the sense that the term is unfortunately applied to people. Almost all the dogs in whom I have seen senile cataracts were alert, steady, and had all their "wits" about them.

The cataract of advancing years usually begins at about the age of nine or ten. The white or yellow-white opaque area may start centrally in the same area as nuclear sclerosis or peripherally in all directions, which is the more common type in senior canines. Some develop rapidly to obscure vision totally, but the majority progress rather slowly over a period of many months to years. These opacities generally occur in both eyes at more or less the same rate. It is possible, however, for a cataract to develop only in one eye.

As explained above, it is not necessary to do anything about cataracts, nor should they cause you undue concern, unless they cause secondary problems such as glaucoma. For such dogs, as well as the rare one who is unable to adjust to blindness in a new or old environment, the dog who must be able to see for some individually urgent reason—or for one whose owner can't cope with the idea of having a blind dog—cataracts *can* be removed.

There are no effective medical treatments for cataracts, but the advanced surgical techniques available today, including a freezing method known as cryosurgery, make such operations quite safe and practical in the proper hands. Many veterinarians who have a special interest in eye diseases will have developed the necessary skills to perform cataract extraction and are doing it routinely. In lieu of such skills, your veterinarian will refer you to another colleague who can do this surgery or, where available, to a Board-certified veterinary opthalmologist.

A complete examination of the entire eye must be done first to assure that the only problem with vision is the obstructing cataract. If there is visual deficit anywhere else in the eye, removing the cataract would not restore sight, and the surgery will not be done. Not all cataract operations are successful, but the failure rate is very low.

When he comes home from the hospital after the operation, your dog's feet may be bandaged, or he may be wearing a hood-like collar to prevent him from rubbing at his eyes while they are healing. You may also be given medications to put in the eyes and will probably be advised to keep him in subdued light for a number of days. Your dog will have few, if any, of the postoperative problems people have. He will not need thick eyeglasses and so on. Remember, he doesn't have to read a newspaper or sign a check. After a short period of adjustment to having light enter his eyes once more, your dog will be able to distinguish light from darkness and see large or moving objects easily. There may be some lack of clarity with small or stationary objects. But *your dog can see again*, and that is what matters most.

There are two other types of cataracts which I would like briefly to mention. Injury to, or around, the eye can alter the health of the lens and produce an opacity. This is less likely to occur in older dogs than in the bouncy, hyperactive or aggressive younger ones. The second type is the so-called diabetic cataract, which *may* develop in dogs with diabetes mellitus. Both types can be handled surgically provided all underlying causes and complications have been corrected.

Glaucoma

Just as cataracts are not limited to the older canine, so can glaucoma develop at any and all ages. In the dog, this latter disorder of the eye is due to interference with the flow and drainage of aqueous humor, the fluid inside the eyeball, which results in a progressively increasing fluid pressure in the affected eye. It might be likened to an overinflated soccer ball in which extreme pressures are exerted equally in all directions. In the eye, the optic nerve, which transmits light impulses to the brain, is extremely vulnerable to injury by the increased pressure, so that this often results in a functional loss of vision.

The majority of glaucoma cases seen in mature and aging dogs are the result of some other primary eye problem such as cataracts, dislocation of the lens, foreign objects or bleeding inside the eye, eye infections, and certain tumors. Since there can be so many causes, the symptoms similarly will be quite variable. Some that are common to many patients include an abnormal or excessive dilatation of the pupil, distention of the veins of the sclera (the white of the eye), haziness or clouding of the cornea (the clear "window" at the front of the eye), and eye pain. The longer glaucoma exists, the greater will be the intensity of these signs. Depending on the specific cause, it may occur in one or both eyes.

A double-pronged approach is needed, in that the underlying cause must be found and corrected quickly while the excessive fluid pressure is reduced by medication, eye surgery, or a combination of both. Early and accurate diagnosis is essential to prevent permanent damage to the optic nerve and blindness. Neglected glaucoma can so severely destroy other eye structures as to necessitate the removal of the entire eye.

Your veterinarian will prescribe medication intended to decrease aqueous humor production as well as increase effective drainage. They may be applied directly to the eye or given by mouth. They must be given at very frequent intervals over the day, especially the ones put directly in the eye. Because your dog with glaucoma is unable to constrict the pupil, you should avoid bright sunlight and very bright indoor lighting, as this would cause him considerable discomfort. As the eye pressure is reduced, most of the pupil's function will return. Frequent examinations may be needed to assess the changing eye conditions and alter medications accordingly. Many glaucoma patients can thus be controlled successfully all their lives.

Some cases do become resistant, or at least less responsive, to medical treatment, and surgery will have to be considered. The goal of the operation is to provide a new channel through which the eye fluid can drain, thus keeping the pressure down. As with cataract removal, this surgery should only be done by a family veterinarian thoroughly experienced in eye surgery or by a veterinary ophthalmologist. You can be sure your doctor will advise you appropriately, as his prime concern is with what is best for your dog.

Once in a while, an eye will respond to neither medication nor surgery, or else pressure develops so rapidly as to threaten rupture of the eyeball. Such an eye must be totally removed because of the severe pain and the danger of imminent rupture. Following enucleation (eyeball removal), healing is fairly rapid, with minimal discomfort to your dog, when he returns home. Short-term medication effectively controls this discomfort. Carefully done, the cosmetic appearance after enucleation is hardly noticeable to strangers at a distance. Your dog will rarely act any differently than he would with two eyes. Of course, you know the eye is gone, but so is your dog's pain and the threat to his life.

Keratoconjunctivitis sicca or "Dry Eye"

Normal tears lubricate and carry nutrition to the cornea, and protect the eye by diluting and washing away any foreign materials that get into it. Any reduction in the amount of tears, which are produced in the lacrimal glands of each eye, will result in varying degrees of drying of the eye. This condition is observed more frequently in older dogs, particularly the miniature poodle, pug, and cocker spaniel, and can occur in one or both eyes.

When tear secretion is sufficiently reduced, the cornea develops a dull appearance, and the conjunctiva, the pink lining of the eyelids, becomes red and swollen. The resultant unpleasant eye discharge is sticky, stringy, and difficult to wipe away. The eyelids are kept partially closed, and ulcers often develop on the cornea. Neglected, keratoconjunctivitis sicca will cause blindness.

It appears that the reduced tear secretion is due to damage to the nerves that stimulate the lacrimal glands. In older canines, this can be caused by physical injury about the head, tumors in or around those nerves, or by a secondary reaction to serious weakening diseases like uterine infection, chronic kidney disease, and severe metabolic disorders. It is also possible for chronic eye irritations to make the glands unresponsive to normal nerve stimulation.

Treatments vary with cause, but all are directed at supplying the necessary moisture to the eye in one way or another. In mild cases, artificial tears instilled into the eye four to six times a day may be all that is needed. If the nerves are still partially functional, the application several times daily of a drug to stimulate tear secretion may be advised. This same drug can be given by mouth but requires extra care as it is potentially toxic in its oral form. Antibiotic and steroid drops or ointments are frequently used as well. Should these medications, alone or in combination, succeed in producing an adequate tear flow they will have to be continued indefinitely as "dry eye" rarely improves. This is easy to do but does require a fairly strict adherence to the time intervals advised in order to avoid even temporary drying. An occasional case will respond to the use of a long-lasting eye lubricant which can be applied only two or three times over the twenty-four hour day.

Some dogs with this tear disorder will not respond to any medical therapy, and when three or four weeks of such attempts bring no results, such pets should be considered for surgery. An operation has been developed fairly recently which has a high success rate, and I recommend it in most cases when medical treatment fails. The duct of the parotid salivary gland, one of several salivary glands on each side of the face, is surgically transplanted to the affected eye in such a way that the secretions from the gland flow over the eye as tears would, thus lubricating and protecting the cornea. After such an operation, little, if any, medication is needed. One minor problem is that the parotid gland will be stimulated whenever your dog eats, and excess "tears" may appear in the affected eye. These can of course be readily wiped away. However, your dog may become a topic of neighborhood conversation as the dog who cries when he eats!

Tumors

All structures within, on, or around the eye are capable of developing tumors, either benign or malignant. They may be primary in the eye and spread to other organs, such as malignant melanoma which spreads to the lungs; or they can develop secondarily in the eye by metastasis from other organs, like mammary gland adenocarcinoma, which is the most common source of eye tumor originating in other organs. Although benign eye growths do occur, the percentage of malignancies is considerably higher. Local surgery, chemotherapy, and radiation therapy each may be useful, but in many cases it is necessary to remove the entire eye. Diagnosis and, even more so, prognosis is quite difficult, and should be made by a veterinary ophthalmologist in most cases. Fortunately for your aging dog, there is no increased incidence with age. If she hasn't had any eye tumors so far, she is no more likely to get them during her senior years.

The eyelids behave differently, however, and there is a significant increase in tumors of these structures as your dog grows old. In fact, eyelid tumors are extremely frequent in geriatric dogs. Fortunately, most of them are benign, and early surgical removal solves the whole problem. The irritation and inflammation of the eye, which is what will prompt you to have the eye examined, clear up rapidly. However, if therapy is delayed, a chronic irritation can result which may not clear up after surgery. Even if the tumor is malignant, early removal before it metastasizes often brings a permanent cure. It is usually not possible for your veterinarian to tell whether the tumor is benign or malignant just by looking at it, so he will submit it to a pathologist for identification. If the report indicates it is benign, everyone breathes a sigh of relief. A report of malignancy may bring a recommendation for chemotherapy, radiation therapy, or additional surgery.

The key to the treatment of eye tumors, like tumors anywhere in the body, is early diagnosis. The maxim "he who hesitates is lost" is all too true in too many cases. Your dog has only two eyes—don't jeopardize them. *Any* eye irritation or unusual discharge which lasts for more than forty-eight hours should be examined by your veterinarian.

11
The Musculoskeletal System

The skeleton has been likened to a frame upon and from which the rest of the body hangs, and this is almost literally true. But it does more than just prevent the body from collapsing in a heap. It also provides protection to certain vital but vulnerable organs—the skull shielding the brain and the rib cage sheltering the heart and lungs. The bones of the skeleton serve as points of attachment for muscle tendons, and it is through the contraction of these muscles that walking and other movements are made possible. Bones and muscles function as a *team* for mobility, and disorders in one usually affect the other. They are, therefore, considered as a single system.

Muscle Atrophy

The muscles of most aged mammals lose much of their strength and actually decrease in size with each advancing year. This is a normal part of the aging process and is to be expected. However, there are two as yet poorly understood muscle disorders which at first may look like normal aging weakness. In one the dog develops weakness in the leg muscles during periods of exercise or other physical stress, may fall down briefly, seem to recover, get up for a short time only to fall down again. This is often seen in *polymyositis*, a disease which causes inflammation of any or all muscles in the body. Those on top of the head are frequently shrunken and, like any of the affected muscles, may be painful to the touch. When resting and relaxed the dog will appear to be perfectly normal.

Polymyositis occurs mostly in late middle age and early old age, the most common of its several possible causes appearing to be a defect in the dog's immune mechanism. Treatment with corticosteroids is quite successful despite the often alarming appearance of the dog. Occasionally the muscles of the esophagus are affected, making swallowing difficult, but even these respond. Dogs with an affected esophagus do require longer treatment and sometimes hospitalization.

Muscular dystrophy, the second disorder, occurs mainly in older dogs, bears some similarity to muscular dystrophy in people, and has a cause as yet unknown. Affected dogs develop a stiff gait as the muscles become progressively weaker and smaller in size. There is nothing we know of which will stop the deterioration or cure the disease. Treatment is palliative, trying to keep the patient as comfortable as possible, and is based on your dog's individual symptoms.

Degenerative Joint Disease (Osteoarthritis, Arthritis)

Noninfectious osteoarthritis is the commonest form of joint disease in the aging dog, a situation not too different from that in humans. The disease is progressive and causes few, if any, noticeable symptoms in the early stages. It is not uncommon for a veterinarian to discover the existence of degenerative joint disease or its predisposing causes during a routine checkup.

Primary arthritis develops from the normal wear and tear of a joint with time and age. While seen occasionally in very old dogs, it is not the commonly observed arthritis that it is in people. The bulk of aging dog arthritis cases are secondary to disorders which happened or started earlier in life. The following are just a few of the many such disorders:

• Obesity in any breed but especially in the large and giant breeds.

• Mechanical trauma such as falls and jumping mishaps.

• Torn ligaments in any joint but especially the stifle joint in toy or miniature poodles.

• Chronic dislocating patella (slipped knee cap), most common in toy breeds.

• Osteochondritis dissecans, a disease of young dogs.

• Hip dysplasia.

• Legge-Calve-Perthes disease, a hip joint disorder common in young toy breeds.

Detecting and correcting to the fullest possible extent any such conditions which can lead to arthritis will delay the timetable of its disabling course and may prevent it entirely.

One of the earliest signs of osteoarthritis is a slight limp or stiffness. There may be pain when the joint is touched or when it is bent. Swelling is uncommon, as are redness and a warm feeling unless there is an infection present in addition to the degenerative process. With the passage of time, the pain and lameness become more noticeable, and the ability to flex and extend the joint is increasingly limited. Even though his examination points to osteoarthritis, your veterinarian will want to x-ray the affected area to rule out other possible causes such as bone tumors. If there is swelling or redness, he may also take a sample of the fluid within the joint space to check for any infection.

No one can cure degenerative joint disease, but with your cooperation your dog can be made rather comfortable and afforded a satisfactory degree of joint function for several years. The first and obvious step is to correct any still existing predisposing causes. The obese dog must be reduced as rapidly as is safe to do. Even the normal dog should take some weight off to reduce the force being applied to the sick joint or joints. All strenuous and unnecessary exercise should be stopped. Limited, normal walking should be encouraged, however, to keep the joint movable. Too much rest or inactivity will allow the joint to become even stiffer. Try to eliminate all very smooth surfaces on which your dog might slip.

In painful acute flareups, your dog may be given corticosteroid injections for a short time to relieve the severe discomfort. After that, he will most likely be treated by you at home with aspirin, in one form or another, given with some food three or four times a day in carefully calculated doses. As the degeneration of the joint progresses over months and years, it may be necessary to increase the dose. This should not be done without discussing it with your veterinarian first. Aspirin in high doses can be dangerous and must be used with caution. In some fortunate cases it may be possible to actually reduce the dose, but it is unlikely that it could be totally discontinued. Sometimes corticosteroids are combined with aspirin or may be used alone later when aspirin is no longer effective at a safe dose. There are other drugs which may also occasionally be prescribed.

In certain cases of osteoarthritis, it may be advisable to arthrodese (surgically fuse) the joint surfaces so the joint can no longer move, thus eliminating the source of pain. This cannot be done in every joint. It is used most often in joints of the legs and sometimes in the vertebral column. A certain degree of stiffness and awkward gait will result, but your dog will be free of pain.

The phenomenal advances currently being made in the *total replacement* of severely arthritic crippled joints are having wider acceptance in human medicine. Total hip replacement is now being done with some success in selected canine patients. In the future, the implantation of artificial joints in other disabled parts of a dog's skeleton will almost surely be possible.

Bone Fractures

The bones of aging dogs undergo varying degrees of demineralization and may become brittle. It therefore takes less injury to them to cause a fracture. Slips and falls, from which your dog used to bounce right back, now might easily break a bone. Providing good footing to walk on, avoiding slippery surfaces, and keeping the toenails properly trimmed can help avoid such mishaps.

Because of the reduced state of mineralization, bone fractures in the geriatric dog heal more slowly and may require different or more complicated methods of repair than the same injury in a younger dog. Splints, casts, bone pins, bone plates, and other devices used to immobilize broken bones usually have to be left in place for more extended periods of time.

Geriatric Intervertebral Disc Disease

There are few more pathetic sights than that of a dog pulling himself about by his front legs while the paralyzed hind legs drag limply behind. Yet degeneration of an intervertebral disc at any of several points in the vertebral column can frequently produce such a dog. Disc degeneration is a *normal*, pain-free process which continues throughout most of life, usually without producing illness. In the dachshund, cocker spaniel, poodle, pekingese, beagle, lhasa apso, shih tzu, and similar breeds this degeneration starts early in life and progresses rapidly. Thus when it occurs, the disease is one of the young and the middle years. In most other breeds it starts much later, follows a slowly progressive course, and only occasionally causes disease from late middle age on into old age.

Located between every vertebra in your dog's back, except the first two in the neck or the vertebrae in the tail, these discs act as shock absorbers. They uniformly distribute the pressures applied to them whenever the back is bent, turned, or twisted. With a tough outer capsule and a soft semi-fluid center, they are uniquely equipped to do their job. As degeneration ensues, the soft center becomes semisolid and the capsule weakened; the vertebral pressures are no longer evenly distributed, and the shock absorbers cannot function properly. With time, the capsule may develop a particularly weak spot and start to bulge at that point. If the protrusion happens to be in an upward direction, pressure is put on the spinal cord, which lies just above the disc; and pain, leg weakness, or paralysis can occur. The discs which cause such symptoms most frequently are the secnd and third ones in the neck and those in the middle of the back where the chest joins the lower back. However, disc disease can and does develop in any of the intervertebral discs in the entire spinal column.

It should be apparent that almost any undue pressures on the aging discs could cause protrusions. Your older dog should be kept from violent jumping, especially up and down on his hind

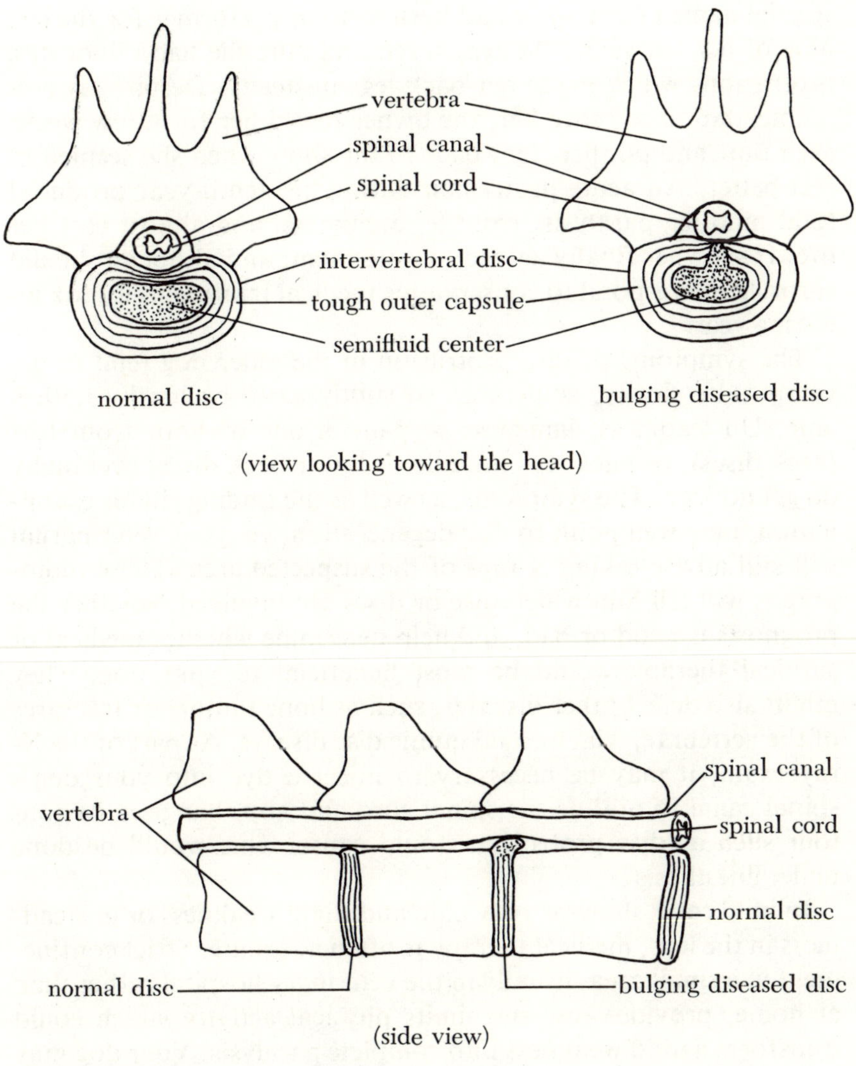

Healthy and diseased intervertebral discs. Note the bulging semifluid center of the diseased disc compressing the spinal cord upward against the vertebra.

legs. Games and other activities that require him to run fast and then suddenly stop or turn should be avoided. Limited and controlled exercise, as described elsewhere in this book, will be less likely to cause a disc problem. I am reminded of a part cocker spaniel named Cheri who had been a circus performer for the last nine of her ten years. At ages seven and nine she had minor disc protrusions which made her back legs unsteady. Despite my recommendation to retire her, the owner rested her for a few weeks each time and put her right back in the show when she seemed to feel better. An acute protrusion during her tenth year produced total hind leg paralysis, front leg weakness, and almost cost her life. Her owner finally agreed to retirement, and although she did surprisingly respond to conservative medical treatment, it took almost a year.

The symptoms of disc protrusion in the older dog tend to develop quite slowly, sometimes so subtly as to be hardly noticeable. Unsteadiness, lameness or pain in one or both front legs (neck discs), or back legs (middle or lower back discs) eventually do get noticed. The symptoms, as well as the findings in his examination, may well point to disc degeneration, yet your veterinarian will still advise taking X rays of the suspected area. These radiographs will tell him which disc or discs are involved, whether the prognosis is good or bad, and help determine whether medical or surgical therapy would be most beneficial to your dog. They might also detect other diseases, such as bone tumors or fractures of the vertebrae, which could mimic disc disease. As part of the X-ray exam, it may be necessary to inject a dye into your dog's spinal canal to outline the spinal cord and any change in its contour such as disc protrusion would cause. This would be done under anesthesia.

In mild cases showing only pain and slight weakness or unsteadiness in the legs, medical therapy is often adequate. Strict confinement in a small area, usually in the veterinary hospital rather than at home, provides rest and limits physical activity which could transform a mild weakness into complete paralysis. Your dog may be given muscle relaxants to reduce the spasms adjacent to the affected discs or antiinflammatory drugs to reduce local inflammation. Medication to reduce the pain will also be given, but only in doses sufficient to lower the level of pain, not completely eliminate it. The slight discomfort that remains will help keep your dog inactive. If all the pain were relieved, he might try to be normally active and possibly cause additional disc and spinal cord injury. Varying with each individual dog, response and healing will be under way in two to three weeks, and your dog will be sent home with instructions for either continued confinement or very limited activity. Oral medications may also be prescribed for home use.

The more severe cases of this degenerative disease, in which there is moderate to complete paralysis, severe pain, or loss of bladder or bowel function, are usually best treated by surgical means. There are two types of operations currently in use, but both have the same goal—to relieve the pressure of the protruding discs on the spinal cord. In one technique, a small opening is made in the *underside* of the offending disc, and the semisolid material in it is scooped out, removing the source of the protrusion. The other type of surgery, called decompression, removes various sections of the bony vertebra *above* the spinal cord at the affected site, allowing the cord room in the canal to move away from the protruding disc beneath it.

The success of either operation is inversely proportional to the duration of disease. The longer the spinal cord is under pressure, the greater the chance that it will be permanently damaged and the outcome unsuccessful. You should appreciate that the decision to treat medically or surgically is often not an easy one for your veterinarian to make. Either way has its potential dangers, and many factors other than the disc disease must also be weighed in the geriatric dog. Failing kidneys and advanced heart disease would not make her a good candidate for surgery, and a medical approach might be the choice of necessity, even though it could be less successful in terms of recovery of normal spinal cord function.

When I was in veterinary college, disc surgery was still in its infancy and considered a very dangerous operation. With research, advancement and refinement of neurosurgical methods, especially during the past decade, such operations have become much safer and have significantly increased the number of successful recoveries.

Your part in the continuing care and therapy following surgery is vital to the eventual success we all hope for. Recovery is *very slow* and will require every drop of your patience and cooperation. If your dog lost control over urination before surgery, she may not start regaining it for two or three weeks. You will be taught how to empty her bladder, twice every day, by gently squeezing the back of her abdomen, in order to prevent urinary infections or damage to her aging kidneys. Bowel control may also have been lost and will require periodic enemas. Of course, it goes without saying that you must keep her clean by brushing and washing with a damp cloth, and the area of her confinement must have a soft surface to prevent "bed sores."

The return of your dog's ability to stand up effectively, and eventually to walk, can take a *long time.* While it occasionally may be as short as three or four weeks, it is far more likely to be three or four months and even longer. Various forms of physiotherapy may be advised—whirlpool baths, sitz baths, and massaging affected muscles—to avoid shriveling of unused muscles and to stimulate blood supply and nerve function in the affected limbs. Exercise carts can be made or purchased which will support

Dog with back leg paralysis in an orthopedic cart. *Courtesy of K-9 Carts.*

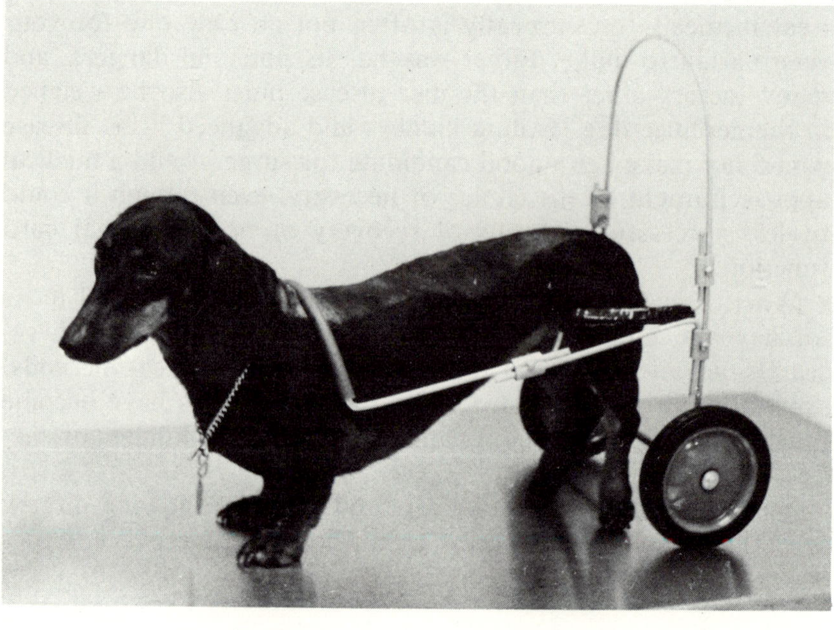

the hind quarters, allowing your dog to walk using her front legs, without the rear ones dragging on the ground. As some control returns, she will be able to paddle her back legs while in such a cart thereby strengthening them further. Most dogs adjust readily to carts and learn to get around their environment with little difficulty. For the occasional dog who does not respond at all to either medical or surgical treatment and is left permanently paralyzed in the back legs, these orthopedic carts along with good nursing care from you can make it possible for her to continue a moderately normal and healthy life.

Goldie had her first problem with an intervertebral disc when she was six years old. She had been chasing after a ball, when she suddenly stopped, screamed momentarily, but then seemed all right. A few minutes later, her hind quarters began to sway. Physical and radiographic examinations showed that two discs in the lower back of this golden retriever were protruding slightly. Since she was already standing much steadier at that point, oral medication and rest at home were prescribed, and three weeks of this brought complete recovery. It was not until two and a half years later that the same thing occurred again, but this time she collapsed on both back legs and couldn't stand at all. Paralysis was total, and she could feel nothing in the back legs.

X rays showed a ruptured disc in the middle of her back. Goldie was referred to a veterinary orthopedic surgeon for corrective surgery that very day. The operation went well, but a week later she still couldn't stand or urinate, although she was regaining some bowel control. When she went home, her owners learned to empty the bladder by pressing on it through the abdominal wall. After four weeks, there was still no improvement, the owners were advised that there might never be any, and she was fitted for an exercise cart. These people would not be discouraged, however, and continued medication, physiotherapy, including whirlpool baths and muscle massage, and endless amounts of TLC (tender loving care). Two months after surgery, Goldie started to feel a little sensation in her back feet and made slight voluntary movements with her toes. When the exuberant owners called to tell me about it, I thought the telephone would pop right off the wall, they were so excited.

From that point on, improvement continued but disconcertingly slowly. Nevertheless, the owners stayed with it! Three months later, I got another excited call. "Goldie just urinated by herself on the living room floor!" The people were so overjoyed they didn't mind mopping up after her for another two weeks, until Goldie was able to control her bladder well enough to urinate outdoors. One year after surgery she still walked with a wobble but she *walked.* It was almost eighteen months before everything returned to normal except for a barely noticeable limp in the right rear leg. Today only her owners and veterinarians can tell she was once a paraplegic.

Like the paraplegic human paralyzed from the waist down, your dog with intervertebral disc disease can be helped in numerous ways to be reasonably self-sufficient and enjoy life for her remaining years. It will take a great deal of commitment, patience, and love from you—all of which, I'm sure, will be there when needed—although nothing you will have to do will be inordinately difficult.

12
The Central Nervous System

Fortunately, the aging dog has relatively few disorders of the brain and spinal cord associated with the process of growing old. Arteriosclerosis, that bane of human aging and a primary cause of senility, is quite rare in dogs. Hence it is unusual indeed to meet a truly senile dog. Cerebral hemorrhage, also called apoplexy or stroke, is likewise a very infrequent occurrence in the canine.

Rabies is caused by a virus which is attracted specifically to nerve tissue and is transmitted by the bite of a rabid animal. However, there have also been rare reports in recent years of airborne transmission. It has been traditionally believed for centuries that once symptoms of rabies develop, death is inescapable, and because of the hazard to other animals and people, such dogs are euthanized if they have not yet bitten anyone. Recent reports of two human rabies cases which were treated successfully and survived the development of rabid symptoms, if confirmed, may possibly alter the present grim outlook for rabid dogs. With the extremely effective and safe vaccines available today to protect your aging dog, however, there is no excuse for you to ever have to worry about this disease.

Loss of hearing in one or both ears can occur from any of the same causes to be found in younger dogs, such as middle or inner ear infections or chronic throat infections. There does take place, as a result of growing old, a slow loss of hearing which can lead to total deafness. This aging deafness is discussed on pages 12–13 under Normal Changes As Your Dog Ages.

Tumors

Tumors of the brain and spinal cord are seen with relative infrequency in the older dog, the former having a higher incidence in boxers and Boston terriers. Symptoms will vary depending on the actual location and size of the tumor but will often include dullness, staggering, pressing the head against a wall, walking in circles, convulsions, or just weakness in one or more legs. In the hands of a competent veterinary neurosurgeon, many spinal tumors can be removed if detected before permanent damage has been done to the spinal cord. Chemotherapy is sometimes needed for a brief period following such an operation. Brain tumors can only occasionally be removed, as most are inoperable due either to their size or location within the brain.

Such was the case with Pon Pon, a gentle and ever so lovable standard poodle. Within a period of only one week he became suddenly aggressive, growled often at his owner, developed an insatiable appetite, and finally had a severe convulsive seizure. In consultation with a veterinary neurologist, an inoperable brain tumor was diagnosed. Medication controlled the symptoms and improved the dog's behavior for almost a month, then seizures started again, but with increased frequency and severity. Medication was ineffective at any dose and Pon Pon was euthanized.

Seizures (Convulsions)

The sight of a dog in a seizure or convulsion is a frightening thing to behold and demands calm, rapid action on your part to prevent her from injuring herself during the attack. *Do not* try to pick her up or to hold her in any way. She doesn't know what she is doing, doesn't recognize you and may very well bite you severely. If the seizure is causing a running "fit" she will race around uncontrollably. There is little you can do other than try to confine her to the room she is in. Should the convulsion cause her to collapse and thrash about, move her away from walls and furniture so she will not hit herself against them. Bunch up a *heavy* blanket, drop it next to her and, with a *long* stick against the bunched-up blanket, push her to the most open, uncluttered part of the room. An old-fashioned push broom, dust mop, floor waxer, or even vacuum cleaner can safely be used for this purpose. Try to confine her to that area by placing more blankets and pillows around her. She may urinate, defecate, or both during the convulsion.

Most seizures last for only a minute or two, some only a few seconds. But it seems like an eternity when you are witnessing it. When the episode is over, *do not* go to pet your dog. She is frightened and still may behave erratically and bite. Talk to her in quiet calming tones of reassurance, and especially use her name if she normally would be responsive to it. She will pant rapidly for a while and her tongue and gums may be fiery red until she relaxes. When she responds to her name, you can reasonably assume that she is most likely back to herself again. *Cautiously* put on her collar and leash, all the while talking soothingly to her. Then phone your veterinarian for an appointment and specific instructions on how to transport your dog to the clinic, as these will vary with what the doctor believes may have caused the convulsion.

Seizures originating in the nervous system of the geriatric dog can be caused by the above-mentioned brain and spinal cord tumors or by epilepsy. It is unusual, though possible, for epilepsy to develop late in life. If your dog is an epileptic, you have probably already lived several years with the disorder and know that it can be fairly well controlled with any of several different drugs or combinations of them, and that your dog can lead an otherwise normal life in between the infrequent seizures. You may also know that maintaining continued control can require, with the passage of months and years, increasing dosages of the same drugs or changing to different ones. Seizures resulting from inoperable spinal cord or brain tumors can sometimes be controlled by these same drugs but usually for only short periods of time, after which all medications are ineffective.

Not all convulsions and seizures result from disease in the nervous system. Certain forms of liver or heart disease, diabetes mellitus, adrenal gland insufficiency, several poisons, as well as the viruses of rabies and distemper, can all cause various types of nervous symptoms including convulsions or seizures. An accurate history, along with the results of regular periodic examinations in your dog's medical records, will assist your veterinarian in the differentiation of the possible causes of your dog's seizure.

Although disease of the intervertebral disc can result in damage to the spinal cord, this disorder is discussed under disorders of the musculoskeletal system on page 182.

13
Infectious Diseases

There are no known infectious diseases peculiar only to aging dogs. Nevertheless, canine distemper, infectious canine hepatitis, leptospirosis, and rabies are of concern to the older dog. These diseases are no respecters of age. They can and do occur at any age! Because immune mechanisms and natural resistance are often reduced in old age, the geriatric dog may be just as susceptible to these diseases as a puppy. Booster vaccinations given at the proper intervals with appropriate vaccines will protect your aging dog.

I first met Rufus six days after he had been taken in as a stray from the streets of New York City. I estimated him to be seven weeks old, and he was showing classical signs of canine distemper. The owner chose not to treat the puppy and took him to a humane society shelter. The following week, this same gentleman called to say he thought his dog had distemper. I thought to myself, "Didn't he give the puppy to the shelter?" And then, "Maybe he adopted another one." Neither! He had neglected to inform me during his first visit, but did so now with obvious pride, that he also owned an eleven-year-old Chihuahua named Snipe who "almost never goes out of the house, hasn't been to a veterinarian in ten years, and is in the peak of health.'' That is, until this particular morning. Upon examining Snipe, I had to confirm the owner's diagnosis of distemper, obviously caught from Rufus.

This gentleman had been convinced that distemper immunity was ''permanent'' and booster vaccines were totally unnecessary. In fact, he admitted he truly believed that veterinarians recommended such boosters only in order to add to their income. Well, Snipe survived and was cured after many weeks of treatment, heartache, anxiety, and expense—all of which could so easily have been prevented. Other older dogs I have known with similar histories were not so lucky and either died or were left with serious impairments.

14
Cancer and Cancer Therapy

Your dog has been diagnosed by your veterinarian as having cancer. After the initial shock or panic has worn off, and the doctor has tried to answer your questions of "How?" and "Why?," you will want to know what kind of future lies ahead of your aging canine and "how much time does he have left?" The answer to the latter question can only be an educated guess as no two tumors, be they benign or malignant, or even of the identical type, act exactly the same way—not even within the same dog. Some tumors are more highly malignant than others and damage more rapidly. "Time left" for these tumors has been suggested in the sections where the specific tumors are discussed.

As much of the tumor as is possible will be removed surgically. If it is an isolated mass and can be taken out "clean," the chances for long-time survival is good. On the other hand, even if it has deeply infiltrated surrounding tissue, surgery may still be done to reduce the volume of cancerous cells in the body and help make additional nonsurgical therapies more effective. Chemotherapy, radiation therapy, immunotherapy, or various combinations of them will control many tumors and reduce some but because of side effects may have to be discontinued for short periods. Eventually they may have to be stopped altogether.

Regardless of the type of cancer treatment undertaken, it will require frequent and continuing visits to your veterinarian, not only for therapy, but for medical checkups, to be sure that your dog's system is coping adequately with the stress of the disease *and* the treatments. Most cancer patients can be made quite comfortable and are able to live fairly normal lives for as long as therapy is effective. However, since cancer generally is an ailment of aged dogs, there are likely to be other disease processes going on, particularly of the heart, kidneys, and liver, which may alter the effectiveness of cancer therapy or otherwise reduce the "time left." Occasionally such a dog's cancer may be so advanced and widespread that any cancer treatment might adversely affect a failing heart or other organs, and your veterinarian will advise against treatment of the tumor. Instead, your dog will be kept symptomatically comfortable until pain or other discomfort no longer responds to medication. It is then time for euthanasia.

What causes cancer? That question was asked as soon as the word cancer was coined and is still being asked today, but with a second question, Why? Why do the many causes of cancer of which we are now aware produce cancerous growths under certain conditions in certain parts of the body and not under others or elsewhere? Most research presently under way is directed toward answering that second question. Among the known causes of cancer are:

- Viruses—such as the leukemia virus in cats.
- Radiant energy—sunlight can cause skin cancer.
- Chemicals—hardly a day goes by that we don't hear about another food additive or other chemical that is believed to be carcinogenic.
- Genetic predisposition—boxers and the giant breed of dogs have an inordinately high incidence of certain types of tumors.
- Hormone association—the dog spayed when young is far less likely to develop breast cancer than one spayed later or not at all; prostatic cancer can be controlled by castration; perianal gland tumors, common in males, are almost never seen in the female dog.

Why does one Great Dane develop bone cancer and another not? Why does one dog develop a brain tumor or breast cancer and another one doesn't? Why? Why? Why? The question is still unanswered, but the search for answers continues among veterinarian, physician, and science research teams in this country, England, Sweden, Japan, and the Soviet Union, among many others throughout the world. The answers, I believe, are in the immediately foreseeable future, and I urge you to contribute to the support of cancer research in any way you can. Your family veterinarian can direct you to research programs working specifically on dog cancer.

It has been said many times over in this book, in the press, on TV, virtually everywhere, that early diagnosis is the key to the successful treatment or control of cancer. Why then, do some dog owners choose to ignore the lumps and bumps on the outside of their dog's body, the breast or testicle that is obviously getting bigger, the steady loss of weight in spite of a ravenous appetite, the gums that are getting thicker and suddenly pigmented, or the leg which is getting thicker than its opposite mate? I suppose many people, dog owners or not, are afraid to find out the truth and just hope "it will go away." But it rarely ever does! *Now* is the time for those abnormalities to be examined and, whenever possible, biopsied. The pathologist's report may bring the happy news of a benign tumor, which can easily be removed or treated, or perhaps of no tumor at all. Even if the report is one of a malignancy, early treatment still offers the best chance for complete cure or at least a prolonged period of control.

Surgery

The best way to get rid of something offensive is to remove it completely. Complete surgical excision is the most effective method of getting rid of a cancer, if it is operable and has not spread. The smaller the tumor, the more likely it can be totally cut out along with enough healthy surrounding tissue to be sure no cancer cells are left behind. Larger ones are mechanically more difficult to remove, often damage surrounding organs, and—the greatest danger—may have metastasized to other parts of the body. In such cases or when the tumor cannot be operated at all, other methods of treatment are available.

Cryosurgery

Tumors of the mouth, the skin covering the paws and tail, and of the anus are often mechanically difficult to remove by conventional surgery with a scalpel. A method developed a long time ago, forgotten for many years but brought to the fore again in the past decade, cryosurgery freezes and kills the tumor. As the frozen tumor thaws out, the dead tissues slowly disintegrate. It is a rather messy and smelly process, of one to several weeks duration, depending on the size and depth, but it does get rid of the tumor. An additional advantage is that it requires less anesthesia, a definite plus in the geriatric dog, and sometimes can be done with only sedation and a local anesthetic.

Chemotherapy

It has been said somewhere that out of every evil comes some good, and out of the horrors of World War II came the discovery that certain types of drugs could kill cancer cells. Since then other drugs have been developed or found to have anticancer activity. They are most effective when the tumor cells are actively growing and less so during those cell's resting stages, hence the frequently seen variation in response to treatment. There are almost two dozen anticancer drugs currently available, and although a single drug may be used alone in some instances, it is more likely your veterinarian will use a combination of two or more to gain the advantages of each while reducing the individual undesirable side effects.

The majority of these drugs cannot distinguish an actively growing cancer cell from an actively growing normal cell, so they often kill healthy cells during therapy. The resulting side effects may include vomiting, diarrhea, loss of appetite, loss of hair, anemia, and the destruction of white blood cells. It is essential that your dog be monitored for these signs of toxicity by means of a physical exam and blood tests done once a week in most cases. In between visits, you must also watch carefully for any abnormal signs and report them immediately to your doctor. Should mild toxic signs develop, the drug dose may be reduced until the signs subside, but severe toxicity will require complete withdrawal of therapy and possibly the administration of supportive treatment for the toxic symptoms. During this withdrawal period the cancer cells will begin to grow again.

As more is being learned about the safer and more effective use of chemotherapy in the treatment of cancer, successful remission of many kinds of tumors, for one to two years, is being achieved. For a dog twelve or fourteen years old, that is a significant extension of life expectancy. Other kinds of tumors have been less successfully treated, and remission must be measured in only weeks or months.

Radiation Therapy

Radiation therapy, another method particularly useful in the treatment of tumors of the skin, the perianal glands, and in and around the mouth, may be used in place of surgery or following surgical excision of tumorous tissue. Because of the very high cost of the necessary equipment—an X-ray unit designed for therapy may cost three to five times more than one intended for diagnosis (X-ray pictures)—radiotherapy is usually available only at veterinary colleges, research institutions, or a veterinary radiologist in private specialty practice. There are some smaller hospitals scattered over most areas which do have such equipment, however, and they serve as centers to which other practitioners can refer their patients who need radiation treatment.

As with chemotherapy, radiation destroys both healthy and malignant cells and is the reason the total treatment dose is generally divided into several smaller doses given at intervals which may range from every two or three days up to every two weeks. There are side effects which are difficult to avoid. The commonest is a redness of the skin, which usually clears up after the end of therapy. Loss of hair often accompanies this redness and may be permanent. If hair does regrow, it is usually white in color. The greatest problem in using radiotherapy is that your dog must be anesthetized *each time* to insure that the treatment is applied only to the immediate area of the tumor. The slightest movement by your dog could direct killing radiation at normal tissue and cause serious problems. As we have already discussed the potential problems of anesthesia in the geriatric dog, you can appreciate the additional risks of repeating it at frequent intervals. With the advent of newer and safer anesthetics, however, radiation therapy has been gaining new favor in recent years.

The reddened skin may ooze following treatment and cause your dog to lick or scratch at it. Your veterinarian will prescribe tranquilizers, soothing lotions and ointments, or a restraint collar to keep your dog from reaching the affected area. This problem generally clears up in a couple of weeks, but your veterinarian will want to check him in about a month and again at two- or three-month intervals. If there has been no recurrence after six months, most doctors consider the cancer cured, as it is highly unlikely to recur after that interval. Nevertheless, your dog should be reexamined every six months for the rest of his life just as a precaution.

Immunotherapy

Perhaps the most promising area in the treatment of cancer today is the still young and somewhat experimental field of immunotherapy. This method is an attempt to stimulate the body's own immune mechanisms to produce an immune reaction (antibodies) against the cancer cells. Although it is an extremely complex group of mechanisms, it is in some ways similar to the manner by which distemper vaccine stimulates an antibody response against the distemper virus. So far, the results have been quite variable. Because the procedures are still being researched, your family veterinarian will probably have to refer you to a veterinary oncologist (tumor specialist) for treatment by these methods. For the present, immunotherapy is used in conjunction with surgery, chemotherapy, or radiation therapy but shows promise of some day becoming the primary method of successfully treating a wide variety of cancers.

Lymphosarcoma

Accounting for better than five percent of *all* tumors known to occur in the dog, lymphosarcoma is the commonest malignancy seen in aging dogs, especially those in the eight- to twelve-year range. Its cause is unknown and is relentlessly fatal, but early diagnosis combined with one or more of the therapy modes just described can comfortably prolong life for eight months to a year.

This tumor can develop in any organ or part of the body, and symptoms will naturally depend on the location. If it's in the digestive system, there may be vomiting, prolonged diarrhea, and continuing weight loss despite a good or even ravenous appetite. The liver or spleen may become quite enlarged causing a "big belly." Tumors in the chest can cause coughing and difficult breathing, as can tumefied tonsils. In the skin form, there may be many hard, reddened areas which ulcerate easily. Some dogs show tumor development in one or both eyes, usually in the iris or just under the cornea.

Any or all of these can occur in one dog, but the commonest symptom is enlargement of the lymph nodes located just under the skin on the back of the thighs, the front of the shoulders, and on either side of the throat near the jawbone. Such a dog may appear perfectly normal in all other ways and could misleadingly induce you to ignore the swellings until the tumor spreads further and causes obvious signs of illness.

Biopsy of an enlarged lymph node or suspicious skin will confirm the diagnosis. X-ray studies can confirm additional disease in the chest or abdomen and are essential when there are no external tumors. Blood studies are also helpful, inasmuch as about half of the dogs with lymphosarcoma tumors also have leukemia.

Most cases of lymphosarcoma involve multiple parts of the body, thereby making surgical excision of the tumors impractical, if not impossible. Chemotherapy is the method most often used and initially prednisone, a cortisone-like drug, is the medication generally prescribed. It makes your dog "feel better" and is less dangerous than most other effective drugs. These more toxic drugs may be used later on, or they are sometimes combined with the prednisone right from the beginning of therapy. Radiation treatments and immunotherapy are occasionally used as adjuncts to chemotherapy.

Treatment with all anticancer drugs has undesirable side effects, which limit the time such drugs can be utilized. Stomach and intestinal ulceration and bleeding, sodium and potassium imbalances, urinary bleeding, loss of hair, severe changes in the production of blood cells in the bone marrow, and lowered resistance to infection all occur with considerable regularity and will periodically require temporary withdrawal of the medication. Remission is, therefore, intermittent and almost never complete. But keeping the tumors from getting bigger or even partially diminishing their size can make your dog comfortable for extended periods.

Your dog will be treated as an outpatient once an effective dose has been established, but he will have to be examined and have blood tests done at least twice a month, and not uncommonly every week, to determine when the side effects have reached a dangerous level. Medication will be reduced or suspended until further tests show that it is safe to start again. If the tumors are in the stomach or intestines, a special, easily digested, nonirritating, low fat diet may be recommended. Involvement of different organs may require other special diets. Dogs with coexisting leukemia will probably be given antibiotics, and any dog with lymphosarcoma may need fluid therapy or other supportive treatments to make him comfortable and functional for as long as remission can be secured.

PART THREE
Death

15
Death—When the Time Comes

For every thing there is a season,
and a proper time is for every pursuit under the heavens.
There is a time to be born, and a time to die,
a time to plant, and a time to pluck up what hath been planted.

—Ecclesiastes 3:1, 2

Throughout this book so far we have been examining ways and means of prolonging your dog's natural life and making it as healthy, comfortable, and happy as is humanly possible. Daisy may now be fourteen, sixteen, or maybe even twenty years old. She has had her good days and bad, has had an operation or two, and perhaps has even been brought back from the brink of death through the concerted efforts of you and your family veterinarian. You have done so many little things to make her senior years easier for her, and she has managed to always retain her young dog outlook. You cannot conceive of the idea that she will not always continue to be there when you call to her.

Yet you realistically know that we are all placed on this earth for only a very finite period of time and that eventually what is called death must indeed come. I refer to physical and physiological death—all agree to the occurrence of that aspect. Your own personal beliefs may or may not include other aspects of death which will not be entered into here. Such beliefs may make it easier for you to accept the passing away of your beloved and devoted companion of so many years.

I cannot say, I will not say
That she is dead. She is just away!
With a cheery smile and a wave of
  the hand,
She has wandered into an unknown
  land,
And left us dreaming how very fair
It needs must be, since she lingers
  there.
Think of her still as the same, I
  say:
She is not dead, she is just away.

—James Whitcomb Riley

The end of physical life sometimes comes very suddenly and without any apparent warning.

Trixie is fifteen and a half, has had geriatric checkups every year since she was six and has had no major illnesses. In fact, at her last checkup only two months ago, her veterinarian said that she looked and acted like a five-year-old except for those few gray hairs around her muzzle. And last night she was perky and playful at bedtime—she even brought you her favorite chew toy for you to play with her. There were no sounds heard during the night. Yet Trixie is dead when you wake up this morning. At first you think she is just sleeping deeply, she is so quiet and peacefully relaxed. But soon the truth is apparent—Trixie has passed away in her sleep without any pain, fear, suffering, or prolonged illness. Weep for your loss but be grateful for Trixie's boon of an easy departure from this life. Would that all dogs could die in a like manner.

Poochy has been slowing down for quite some time now. He's had a few serious geriatric ailments but they were successfully treated medically or surgically. Now there have been recurrences or he no longer responds to medication or new illnesses develop which cannot be treated. He is uncomfortable, doesn't want to move about too much, and shows no interest in eating or drinking. You hold Poochy's well-loved head in your hand as you try to finger feed him. Out of his great love for and desire to please you, he tries to lick a little from that friendly finger but doesn't seem to have the energy left to do so. The intravenous feeding and other fluid therapy his doctor gave him yesterday perked him up a bit for a few hours, but he's so much worse today. He's having difficulty controlling his bladder and bowels and has soiled himself with both feces and urine. Now he whimpers on and off as if in pain. Poochy is living, but the *quality of his life leaves much to be desired*.

Taffy has had a serious setback in her most recent illness and has been hospitalized again. Despite standard and even heroic measures by her veterinarian—antibiotics, steroids, fluid therapy, chemotherapy, blood transfusions, radiation therapy, peritoneal dialysis—she continues to get worse. She, too, refuses to eat or drink, becomes incontinent, and is in pain. Taffy is alive, but the *quality of her life leaves much to be desired*.

We have all heard the old adages that "life must go on" or "where there is life there is hope." But is there hope for the hopelessly ill? Must life go on regardless of the quality of that life? There is such a great disparity between living and being kept alive!

Your family veterinarian who has cared for Jiggs for the past twelve of his sixteen years, having examined him thoroughly, performed all the diagnostic tests indicated by his current illness, and carefully and thoughtfully assessed the test results therefrom, says to you those words we each would like never to hear. "I'm truly sorry to have to tell you that Jiggs has a terminal illness. There is nothing we now know that will cure or in any way successfully treat his condition. It is only a matter of time—a few weeks, hopefully a few months, perhaps only a few days."

You sit there stunned, even though you half-expected it, and try to fight back the tears that well up in your eyes. Thousands of images flash through your mind's eye as you recall those myriad times of great joy and happiness brought into your life by that shaggy little fellow you named Jiggs. Funny, you can't even remember why you called him that. But what matter the name, he has given you so much and asks so little in return. As your vision becomes blurred by the stream of tears, you also remember those times that were not so smooth—the difficulty you had housebreaking him, the time he accidentally knocked over and broke your favorite lamp as he chased after a strange cat in the house, and other times when you momentarily had second thoughts about Jiggs. But they are so inconsequential compared to the enormous emotional enrichment he has brought into your life.

After pulling yourself together, your first question might be, "Are you sure, doctor?" "As sure as it is possible to be," comes the answer. Your blood starts to race again, panic is about to take hold, and your next thought could be to take Jiggs to another doctor, and maybe another and another, until you find one who will say what you so desperately want to hear—that Jiggs can be cured. Through all of this, you faintly hear your veterinarian saying, "Because of the seriousness of the diagnosis, perhaps you would like to obtain a second opinion." Aha!, you think, the doctor isn't sure! Quite the contrary—the doctor is very sure. But no conscientious veterinarian considers himself infallible, and because of the extremely serious diagnosis and its imminent consequences, in order to give you *any* possible benefit of doubt, and to help set your mind at ease, he suggests obtaining an independent opinion to either corroborate or refute his.

In each of these cases, your veterinarian has told you there isn't anything further that can be done to cure, treat, or alleviate the suffering that is now developing. Throughout the course of the illness, you have prayed, in whatever form that act takes as a part of your life, for your dog's recovery or at least some improvement. You have looked inward for any possible indication that you may have in some way caused or contributed to your dog's serious problems. But no matter how hard you seek, you cannot find any such evidence! You know deep down you have always done everything you could to make your dog's life healthier and happier, and this is so. You have nothing to feel guilty about! You have not brought about this illness. It is not your doing.

There is a time to be born, and a time to die. . . . The time has come and is *now*!

You and your veterinarian will both want to keep your aging dog alive as long as possible, but each of you may have definite but differing guidelines which could shorten that lifetime. Some dog owners feel that a routine or simple therapy for an older dog is all right, but that heroic treatments or diagnostic procedures should not be undertaken. They may be right, but to these persons I pose the question, "What constitutes an heroic procedure? An electrocardiogram, oxygen chamber, blood transfusion, heart catheterization, peritoneal dialysis, total hip replacement, cardiac pacemaker, X rays, or perhaps an antibiotic injection?" You are surprised by my inclusion of antibiotics? Well, in the immediate pre-World War II years, the administration of penicillin to a human was looked upon as an extremely heroic therapy until the war made it a routine procedure. Before that war, blood transfusion was also considered somewhat heroic. And in the twenty or so years just ahead of us, total organ replacement for dogs will probably become a routine therapy! So what is heroic and what is routine? Your own feelings about medicine, aging, and death will have to define those two words for you.

At the other end of the spectrum are those dog owners who insist upon everything that veterinary medicine can do to keep their aging dog alive. They demand this even if the dog is suffering and can no longer respond to any form of therapy *on its own* but only with aid of respirators, indwelling catheters, repeated dialysis, twenty-four hour intensive care, and indefinite hospitalization.

Happily for the canine, most dog owners fall somewhere in between, being heroic where such actions have a reasonable likelihood of yielding positive results but not indulging their own anxieties or selfishness. Few things make me angrier than the client whose dog is critically and terminally ill, unresponsive to any therapy, and suffering and has the unmitigated gall to say to me while weeping huge tears, "I cannot allow her to die—I love her so much." That client loves herself more than her dog, or she would never allow the untreatable suffering of a pet to continue one moment longer than absolutely necessary!

What about the veterinarian in this matter of maintaining the life of your aged dog? Here too, there is no unanimity of attitude. There may still be a few doctors in practice who will say, "He's just an old dog—what can you expect? He should be put to sleep." There also may be a few who are not capable of performing the particular therapy indicated for your dog's illness or may not have the proper facilities or equipment. The proper thing would be for you to be referred to another veterinarian who is competent in that procedure or has the proper equipment or facility. After all, there are highly skilled veterinarians in small, one-doctor practices as well as in large, multiple-doctor hospitals. However, rather than admit to you (and to himself) that there is something lacking in his skill or hospital, a few doctors may choose to say, "It's incurable. Nothing can be done. He should be destroyed."

Unless this is your first visit to one of these doctors, you will long ago have become aware of these attitudes and will have sought and found another veterinarian. However, if Loki has been a patient of the doctor for many or all of his years, and she has helped you keep Loki happy and comfortable into his senior years or has brought Loki "back from the grave" in the past, you already know that you can accept that doctor's statement of finality—that Loki should be euthanized. *That* doctor has nothing to hide.

What about the doctor whose hospital is the most modern facility in town, with all the latest diagnostic, therapeutic, and supportive equipment available? Suzy has been failing for months and now has an acute episode which brings her to the brink of death as she lapses into a coma. The doctor acknowledges that nothing can be done to make her well but recommends a respirator, artificial kidney machine, external cardiac stimulators, twenty-four hour private veterinary nurses, and so on, because he believes he might be able to keep Suzy alive for a few days—or hours.

Happily again for the canine, almost all veterinarians today fall well within these extremes.

When then, does one "pull the plug?" When does one stop

therapy and allow Poochy to pass away peacefully and naturally? When does one decide to humanely and mercifully terminate Taffy's untreatable pain and suffering by painlessly taking her life—euthanizing her? These are not easy questions for you or any dog owner to answer, even when your dog is seriously ill, and certainly not when your dog isn't even sick. Yet, earnest consideration must be given to the subject and a frank discussion held with your family veterinarian *long before* the moment when a decision has to be made. This is especially true if euthanasia is not within your present realm of consideration.

Most people purchase cemetery plots for themselves and arrange with family members or in their will the details of their own funeral. It is not morbid to think about death while one is feeling well. Nor is it morbid to plan ahead for that painful time when death will come in some form to your beloved dog. At the next geriatric examination, ask your veterinarian about the end of a dog's life. Openly express your feelings about it so the doctor can better understand them and perhaps clarify some of your misunderstandings or misgivings. You will find it much easier to discuss and come to rational decisions while Taffy is in good health than when you are upset and distressed by her pain and suffering.

"What would you do, doctor?" you ask as tears well up in your eyes at the mere thought of Loki ever leaving you. While every veterinarian would like to be able to give you a simple definitive answer, it is rarely possible to do so. It is also unfair. If her advice does not happen to agree with your feelings at the moment, you may feel under pressure to alter those feelings. All your doctor can realistically do for you is to explain in detail what Loki's problems are, what if anything can be done to alleviate them and for how long, whether or not he is in pain or is suffering, and give you an educated estimate of how long he might continue to live. The decision to allow death, or to produce it, is one you must be able to live with. Therefore, the final decision must rest with you, not your doctor, and is one you should not abdicate from making.

> Take time to deliberate; but when the time for action arrives, stop thinking and go in.
>
> —Andrew Jackson

What help then, do you have in making that difficult decision? There are six criteria which should enable you to come to a correct conclusion. *Chronological age, in itself, is never one of them!* All other things being equal, which I grant they often are not, virtually any medical or surgical procedure that can be done for a young dog can be done for an aged dog.

1. Is the condition prolonged, recurring, or getting worse?
2. Is the condition no longer responding to therapy?
3. Is your dog in pain or otherwise physically suffering?
4. Is it no longer possible to alleviate that pain or suffering?
5. If your dog should recover, is he likely to be chronically ill, an invalid, or unable to care for himself as a healthy dog can?
6. If your dog recovers, is he likely no longer to be able to enjoy life, or will he have severe personality changes?

If your answers to all six are "yes," I feel that he should be euthanized so as to stop unnecessary suffering. If your answers to three and four are "no," then perhaps he should be allowed to die naturally, but you must then answer three more questions.

1. Can you provide the necessary care?
2. Will such care so interfere with your own life as to create serious problems for you or your family?
3. Will the cost involved become unbearably expensive?

These last three may be harder to answer accurately, because they require subjective rather than objective determination. Your veterinarian can outline the type of care that will be needed, the amount of time it will involve, whether or not Loki can be left alone and for how long, how frequently office visits will be necessary, what approximate expenses you can expect, and so on. But do you have the physical as well as emotional strength to medicate, feed, and clean Loki? Can you make the time to take him out more frequently, if he isn't paper trained, and to do all the other things required by his illness? Are there others in the family who would help? What happens if you must go away for a few days—is there someone else to take over for you? And finally, how much and for how long can you afford the costs of such care, whether at home or in the hospital?

Jiggs has a terminal illness but research is being done on it at an institution across town. Reports of success are premature but promising. However, more canine cases are needed for testing the new treatment. They cannot assure you that Jiggs will be cured or improved. They will try. But they will not make Jiggs any more uncomfortable, nor will they allow him to suffer. If he does improve, he will be returned to you; otherwise they will euthanize him. You may wish to consider this possibility.

Natural Death

When the end of my life comes I hope it will arrive while I am sleeping and proceed quietly, quickly, and painlessly without waking me up. I wish the same providential release from this life for all who must die, be they two legged, four legged, or no legged.

It may be your good fortune to have an aged dog who has avoided the many ailments seen so often in advancing years; whose quality of life is little different from what it was during her middle years . . . and some morning when you wake up, or some evening when you come home from work, you find Princess cold, rigid, and not breathing. It is even possible that death may come during your presence, although most dogs, sensing some momentous change about to take place (we believe they have no concept of death), will try to seek seclusion by going to another room or crawling under a piece of furniture or into a closet. As the life clock begins to run out, the dog will lie down, usually on its side, breathe very deeply and, as the clock stops, relax all over. The eyes will probably remain open, the mouth relax, and the tongue, by now a dark purple or bluish-gray, may hang loosely from it. If the lower bowel and bladder happen to be full at this time, feces and urine may pass out as the muscular rings which normally keep these organs closed start to relax. These last two occurrences are virtually sure signs of death.

Nevertheless, watch the chest wall carefully to see if there is any up and down movement to indicate she is still able to breathe. A discolored tongue could mean a cardiovascular episode which could be helped by emergency treatment. Put your ear to her chest wall just behind the upper arm at the level of the elbow. Be sure it is quiet in the room and listen for a heartbeat, taking care not to mistake the now rapidly pounding beat of your own heart for that of Princess. If it is indeed death, the body will remain relaxed and warm for some time, depending on the cause of death, before it starts to become stiff—rigor mortis.

McGinty is critically ill but happily is not suffering. He is able to stand and walk slowly with only slight discomfort. There is no difficult breathing nor is there any kind of pain. He can eat if hand fed and eliminates wastes by himself. Although terminal, you have chosen to allow him a natural death. The end will come in a pattern similar to Princess. However, depending on the nature of McGinty's illness, there may be some pain or distress near the end. Your veterinarian will be able to provide oral medication to ease the final discomfort but get this well ahead of the time you'll need it. Don't wait till the last minute and then start running to the doctor's office.

Euthanasia

> Death is a punishment to some, to some a gift, and to many a favor.
>
> —Seneca

Euthanasia is defined as painless peaceful death and is derived from the two Greek words *eu*, meaning well, and *thanatos*, meaning death.

Every day we condone and indirectly authorize, by the purchase of their end products, the killing of all types of animals—beef cattle, hogs, lambs, poultry, and so on—which are not sick or in pain but in fact are actually in the best of health. Some of these killings are painless, but most could hardly be called a peaceful death. This is all done in the name of feeding ourselves. Other animals are killed for their fur, skin, shell, tusks, internal organs, and on and on, almost without end. These deaths are truly killing in the worst sense of that word, often maiming and causing extreme pain before the animal is released from its agony by eventual death.

Can we in good conscience and love for our aged canine friend who is now in uncontrollable pain and suffering, for whom veterinary medicine can offer nothing further to ameliorate it, and who continues to grow worse despite your faith and prayers, allow that affliction to go on unabated? Can you look your distressed dog in the eye and honestly say, "It is better you die in pain naturally than for me to permit you to be killed painlessly and peacefully"? I am unable to understand why so many dog owners are more distressed by an unnatural way of dying than they are by an equally unnatural way of living.

The entire subject of euthanasia tugs at our deepest, innermost feelings, beliefs, and foundations. It is a subject about which most people have very strong opinions and little hesitancy to expound on them to others. It can be a very inflaming subject, filled with fears, anxieties, and guilt feelings derived from the entire scope of human sensibility. No one can decide for you, nor determine the validity or lack of validity of whatever decision you make. Some veterinarians, who believe a dog should be euthanized to end its suffering, may refuse to continue treating such a dog, if you reject euthanasia and will ask you to remove the dog to the care of another doctor whose conscience will allow him to continue therapy. The same veterinarian may just as likely refuse to euthanize a dog for whom there is obvious medical hope simply because it is expedient for the owner to be free of his responsibility to that dog.

J. B., a fourteen-year old miniature poodle, had had no major illnesses during his lifetime. Since the time he was ten the only age-related ailments were a briefly enlarged prostate and increasing nuclear sclerosis. He looked and acted like a dog of eight, and yet his owner presented him to me for euthanasia! In shock I asked the woman, herself in good physical condition, who had lost her husband five months previously, how she could possibly consider such an action. Her response was, "J. B. is deaf and blind, otherwise he's OK. But now that I have so much more time to do things by myself, he's becoming a burden." I suppose I must have turned livid with anger at the thought of this woman wanting to destroy an animal who, by her own and frequent previous admission, had brought so much pleasure to her while her husband was alive. She looked at me as if I were ill, and I suppose I was. I told her I would not be party to a cruel and unwarranted slaughter and showed her the door. A few months later, I was told by another client, a friend of hers, that the woman had immediately taken J. B. to a humane organization, told them he had been sick all his life and they *destroyed him*. This all took place more than a decade ago, yet I still tremble in anger at the thought of it!

You've discussed and deliberated the question and decided that euthanasia is the judicious and merciful alternative to take. Having resolved your own distress in arriving at that decision, you now want to be sure than such an action really is *eu thanatos*, a well death. Your mind is racing again with anxious questions. How is it done? Will Samson be frightened? Can I hold him while it is being done? Should I be present at all? Is it quick? What happens to Samson's body? Will it be experimented with?

The first thing you must do is to sign an authorization for your family veterinarian to perform the euthanasia. Whether your state considers Samson as chattel property or you as his legal guardian, it is necessary for you to give your consent in writing. This is the moment of truth. If you still have any doubts, you should not give your consent. The result of euthanasia is very permanent, and, once done, Samson cannot be brought back to life. It might be difficult at first for some owners to live with the euthanasia of their suffering dog, even though confident they did the proper thing, but to authorize it when one is still uncertain or ambiguous about it would indeed be a heavy burden to live with.

Methods of canine euthanasia can be divided into two main groups—those used in clinical practice, private or otherwise, and those used by many humane societies, dog shelters and similar organizations. The latter groups frequently use either carbon monoxide chambers or decompression chambers to produce unconsciousness followed by death. Because the dogs are already unconscious *before* they are asphyxiated, there is no pain. However, these organizations generally place several animals into the chambers at the same time. The dog's confinement in a strange place can cause anxiety or fear, and the presence of other dogs exhibiting similar responses, will heighten these emotions.

In clinical practice euthanasia is quite another matter. Samson is treated as an individual, and, as such, euthanasia is not allowed to demean the end of his life. Quite to the contrary, it permits him to retain his canine dignity to the very end. The doctor will talk to him quietly, trying to calm and relax Samson, who will be handled gently and with tenderness. An intravenous injection is made, usually into the large vein in either front leg, although any large readily accessible vein may be used. The injected medication causes unconsciousness almost instantly and death within a few seconds. Samson reacts in that first second or two as though he were being anesthetized for an operation. His mind and body relax as if he were falling asleep, hence the origin of the euphemism for euthanasia, "putting a dog to sleep." He may take a few deep breaths, then all is quiet and immobile as life departs from his body. In the event Samson is a dog who always gets excited at the veterinary clinic or is naturally aggressive, the doctor may give him a quick-acting intramuscular sedative or tranquilizer to alleviate the dog's anxieties before administering the euthanizing injection. Either way all will be done to provide a quiet, calm, peaceful, reassuring environment in which to perform this *eu thanatos*.

Should you be present when it is done? This depends on you and your self-control. It is important that you do not display your own distress in front of Samson but rather be supportive and reassuring and, by your own calmness, elicit a similar response in him. To do otherwise might upset, frighten, or even panic your dog. Most veterinarians will not object to you holding your dog, although they may ask that an assistant hold the leg into which the injection will be made. The doctor will explain to you exactly how to hold your dog. For several minutes after Samson is dead there may be a slight twitching of muscle fibers in or under the skin. Don't be upset by these sometimes unsightly movements produced by the briefly delayed death of tissues located at the greatest distances from the heart and brain.

On rare occasions, death may not be instantaneous. The intravenous injection must be pumped by the heart to all tissues and pass through the liver and kidneys before reaching all parts of the body. In some aged dogs with cardiovascular, renal, or hepatic impairment it may take from ten to sixty seconds for death to occur, but relaxation and unconsciousness will still develop very quickly.

Perhaps you do not have adequate self-control to witness your dog's euthanasia. In that instance you will sign the authorization and leave. But you've heard rumors about "experimentation."

How do you know your veterinarian won't experiment on Samson before euthanizing him or, even worse, give him to a research group for experimentation? If you have trusted your family veterinarian with Samson's life all these years, you surely know such anxieties are without basis. Few private practitioners have either the interest or the time to be themselves involved in experimentation of any type. Furthermore, for a doctor to do anything other than euthanize your dog once you have signed such an authorization would be illegal and unethical in most states, subjecting that doctor to severe penalties, including the possible revocation of his license to practice. However, veterinarians recognize that many clients, even the most loyal, may experience such anxieties under the stress of the moment and will ask if you wish to see the body after euthanasia is completed. You can, if you wish, see that your dog is in fact dead.

16
Disposal, Cremation, or Burial

Daisy, Trixie, Poochy, Taffy, Jiggs, Loki, and Samson are now dead—some by natural death, some by peaceful euthanasia. What is to be done with the body? Ideally this has already been decided way back when Daisy was still healthy and you were giving serious thought to the alternatives of natural death or euthanasia. Or else the discussion and decision should have been made before signing the euthanasia consent.

Shall an autopsy be done? Taffy may have been suffering from a rare or unusual ailment. The information to be gained from an autopsy would help your doctor and the veterinary profession as a whole, as well as dogs unknown who will someday develop that same ailment. Death may have come to Trixie without the specific causes being apparent. Both you and the doctor would surely want to know why she died. And then, even though you know the doctor's diagnosis was correct, you might still like to have it confirmed by autopsy just to set your mind at ease. There are, therefore, significant times when an autopsy should be done.

As of this writing, there are no canine organ banks in the United States except for frozen semen banks, which are not quite the same thing. But it will not be very many years before such organ banks, or at least organ transplantation, will be as routine in veterinary surgery as repairing fractures is today. Your veterinarian may know of a dog being treated at another hospital who needs a kidney transplant or an eye replacement. Loki may have a suitable organ for that other dog and you may wish to make it available. If so, you should make your wishes known before euthanasia is done so the transplant organ can be properly prepared and preserved.

Infrequently, a client will have their dog's body preserved by a taxidermist. In this way they try to hold on to the happy memories stimulated by its lifelike presence.

Most of the time the choice is made between disposal of the body by the veterinarian, a private cremation, or burial. If you live in a rural area or otherwise have your own land outside of a large metropolis, you will probably bury Poochy. A heavy plastic bag, cardboard box, or wooden crate can be used to hold the body. The grave should be dug deep enough so wandering animals will not be attracted to dig at the grave site. Three to six feet deep should be adequate, depending upon the type of soil.

Few large cities have animal cemeteries within their boundaries and it is contrary to the health code of most communities to bury an animal on your own or public property within that city. In general, animal cemeteries are located on the fringes of a metropolis. If you have the transportation with which to visit a grave at such cemeteries, then burial is a tender way of remembering a loved canine. Like human cemeteries, most permit headstones and other monuments, while some are completely landscaped with only small markers for each grave. Inasmuch as cemetery plots are fairly expensive, it is important you read the terms of your plot purchase very carefully. Most plots are sold in perpetuity. Some animal cemeteries, however, sell plots for only twenty years or some similar arbitrary period, after which it can be dug up, cleaned, and sold to someone else for another twenty years. In many urban areas there are firms which will make these arrangements for you and conduct a complete funeral service, with organ music, flowers, eulogy, and burial prayers—if you have such a desire.

Almost every community has an animal crematorium. It may be on the premises of, and associated with, an animal hospital, or it may be independently operated. The cremation chamber is thoroughly cleaned after each use so you can be sure the ashes you receive are those of Samson and not some other animal. Private crematoria also may have facilities for you to attend the cremation should you wish to do so. The ashes are then delivered to you in a simple container such as a plastic bag or cardboard box. Special urns, ranging from plain to highly ornate, will be made available should you wish to purchase them. Such urns are then kept at home. Some owners prefer to bury the ashes and know that the physical body of their beloved pet has been converted to the smallest practical remains. City dwellers often bury these ashes surreptitiously in public parks near their homes; others will disperse them into a lake or river. Should you prefer, the crematoria will keep the ashes for you for a specified length of time. The cost of cremation can be substantial and will depend upon the size of your dog.

A frequent choice of the bereaved owner is to have the doctor dispose of the body. It is taken to the incinerator of the community's sanitation department where it is burned with everything else. Next to burying the body yourself, this is the quickest, simplest, and least expensive method of disposal.

Postscript

Another dog?

Of course!

You have lost your beloved canine companion of many years. Death came naturally or was mercifully produced, and he is no more. You are sad, depressed, in emotional pain, and can think only of those former happy days with your deceased dog. "I'll never have another dog! No dog could ever take the place of Buster!" You're absolutely right in your second statement. No dog could nor should be expected to be the same as, or take the place of, any other dog. You will always remember Buster; he was an important part of your life. But a new dog can make his own place in your life, given half a chance, and establish a new and meaningful relationship without in any way detracting from your memories of Buster. It is a rare dog owner who doesn't eventually come to this conclusion, and the sooner it is reached, the better for the person.

There can be situations, however, in which you perhaps should not start with another dog. You may not have the physical stamina often needed to raise a puppy, if you are getting on in years yourself. Perhaps you are nearing retirement and plan to travel a lot or move into a smaller house or an apartment where a dog might not be as welcome. Toilet training, obedience training, two or three times a day walking in all kinds of weather, plus regular exercise may be more than you'd care to cope with, now that you are yourself in your senior years. A puppy will require much more of your time for the first year or so than Buster used to. Are you willing to make that extra time available? A discussion with your veterinarian and perhaps your own physician should help you to make the right decision.

Some dog owners will get a new puppy while Buster is still alive in order to make the transition easier for themselves. Although this may help the people, it is not good for Buster and may not be good for the puppy. You already know that a geriatric dog needs quiet, limited activity, and no stress. A new puppy can be an emotional threat to Buster who may feel that he is already being replaced, as well as sense an instinctive territorial threat. It is certainly a stressful situation for him and could precipitate acute episodes of previously controlled chronic ailments. Your healthy puppy will want to play in ways that may be physically beyond Buster and will feel unaccepted if ignored by the older dog. Now I know of several instances where everything worked out fine, but I feel that these are the exceptions, not the rule. Don't ask Buster to share you with a puppy at a time when he needs you most.

Looking for a new dog won't make you forget Buster, but it will help you to put aside the unhappiness that may have attended Buster's last days. Should the new dog be of the same breed or type as Buster? That depends on your emotional makeup. For some people the same breed will only be a constant visible reminder and will continue an undesirable tie with the past. They will see the new dog only as a new Buster, which will be bad for both them and the dog. For others, the same breed helps them to adjust and accept the new dog. There are no simple answers applicable to everyone, but your family veterinarian has known you and Buster a long time. Discuss the question with her, for she may be in the best position of anyone to help you find the right answer *for you*.

Having chosen the breed or type, do a lot of looking before you do any buying or adopting. The more you look, the more you will really know exactly what you are looking for. Choose a puppy between six and nine weeks of age, if possible, as this is the time when they are best able and ready to make the emotional adjustment from canine siblings to human friend and are less likely to develop emotional problems later on. Be sure you get a written health guarantee for at least forty-eight hours; many reputable breeders and pet shops give two weeks or more. Find out exactly which, if any, injections and worm treatments were given and *when* each was given. Then make an appointment for your veterinarian to examine your new friend, be sure to take along the guarantee and medical information, and take along a fresh stool specimen as well.

And you're off to another long and happy canine-human relationship, perhaps this time for twenty years or more!

Appendix I: Three Love Stories, or, Successfully Living with an Aging Dog

"Hank"—beagle mix—male—
April 1960 to September 18, 1976—age 16½

I saw little of Hank during the first six years of his long life except for regularly scheduled D-H-L and rabies booster vaccinations. Then he began to have "front and rear" problems—infected ears and infected anal sacs. These were to become two of the three hallmarks of his medical history, both recurring periodically throughout the rest of his days. Surgical removal of the anal sacs was advised, but the owner preferred to have them treated whenever necessary rather than have Hank undergo an operation for a problem which was not life-threatening. The ear infections would always respond to initial therapy and then become resistant to it. When it became apparent we would soon run out of new medications, I requested a consultation with a colleague who had a really great "track record" in treating difficult ear problems. Under his care for several months, the ears did improve for longer periods but still continued to be a chronic problem. He recommended a surgical drainage procedure which would significantly improve, but not cure, the disorder. But again Hank's owner declined, resigning himself to daily ear cleaning and regular visits to the veterinarian.

The third hallmark of this dog's medical history was seborrhea, a treatable and usually controllable, but not curable chronic skin disorder. The symptoms started to show up when he was seven and a half, and were vigorously treated with injections, oral medications, antiseborrhea shampoos, and alterations in diet. Initial response was good, but then Hank slowly regressed. When I explained the incurable nature of seborrhea to Hank's owner, he was unhappy about having a third chronic problem, openly questioned my diagnosis and prognosis, and requested another opinion. I suggested that he consult a veterinary dermatologist of his choosing and that my records were available if the doctor wished to have them. Three weeks later, Hank was back in my examination room; the dermatologist having confirmed my unwelcome diagnosis.

Many owners would have given up, but Hank's family loved him very much, even if he did have a rather strong aroma about him from his three chronic disorders. These "dog people" settled down to a routine of regular ear cleaning, anal sac emptying, and frequent shampooing and as they became more adept at their tasks, I had to see Hank less frequently.

Back pain and leg weakness from a slight protrusion of a lower back intervertebral disc occurred when he was ten and a half. Two months of conservative medical treatment at home brought him back to normal. His geriatric exam at twelve disclosed the first signs of alteration in his kidney function and, although there were no physical symptoms, his electrocardiogram showed heart enlargement. Neither required any therapy at the time other than slight changes in his diet.

To "celebrate" the occasion of his fourteenth birthday, Hank developed bronchopneumonia, usually quite serious in aged dogs. But Hank didn't know he was "aged" and responded to treatment as rapidly as a younger dog would. That summer, this spry and playful senior citizen decided to go fishing with his owner and managed to get a fish hook caught in his upper lip (who was fishing for who?). This happened out of town on a weekend, and the owner, unable to find any nearby veterinarians available, called me long distance. As I described over the phone what he should do, the owner step by step succeeded in extracting the hook while Hank stoically stood almost perfectly still. Shortly after his fifteenth birthday, roundworms were discovered in the dog's feces, just as you might expect to find in a puppy. He was treated for them and follow-up fecal exams showed him free of these parasites.

Six months later Hank had a cerebrovascular accident (stroke), an uncommon occurrence in dogs. His head was turned to the side, one front leg was paralyzed, the eyes pulsated rapidly in one direction, and his temperature was below normal. It looked pretty bad for Hank. Other dog owners might have requested euthanasia but not Hank's family. I explained the very grave prognosis, but they felt that they and Hank had been through so much together, that to let him die without trying to help him would be unthinkable. He was put under intensive care including repeated intravenous injections, oxygen, laboratory tests, and constant monitoring. One week later he was able to use that front leg, albeit hesitatingly, and the head tilt was considerably improved. By Christmas, only his owners and I could detect any abnormality in his walking or head posture. Hank was enjoying life and definitely planned on being around for a while!

Right after New Years, the heart enlargement, detected when he was twelve, which remained unchanged for almost four years, became rapidly worse within a period of three days. Digitalization and intense supportive therapy slowly brought the night cough, restlessness, and other symptoms under control. Yet follow-up heart X rays and electrocardiograms showed the heart was continuing to deteriorate. Despite this progressive "wearing out" of his heart and the necessary commensurate changes in medications and their dosages, Hank was quite alert and comfortable right to the end, almost nine months later. He enjoyed eating as always, was bright, responsive, inquisitive, and slept through almost every night. It was during one of his "good night's sleep" that he quietly passed away at home at the age of sixteen and a half.

"Loki"—standard poodle—male—
June 4, 1962, to October 5, 1975—age 13½

Loki started out in life right behind the eight ball by contracting canine distemper as a puppy. Intensive veterinary care, followed with devoted home nursing provided by his owner, Diane, eventually brought Loki back to good health. During the course of his subsequent happy and healthy youth, he had his share of occasional diarrhea, runny eyes, simple skin irritations, poodle ear problems, and sneezing. Minor anal sac difficulties, tonsillitis, and clipper burns (from one of the best groomers in town) were also no strangers to Loki, but he coped with them rather quickly and effectively. This was due largely to Diane's keen ability to know when her dog was the least bit abnormal and her skill in following through on home treatment and good nursing care.

Diane saw to it that Loki received D-H-L and rabies boosters like clockwork, whenever they were due. When he had his first geriatric exam at seven years of age, she did not expect me to find anything wrong. Well, I didn't find very much abnormal. Yet the slight change in kidney function and the very slight enlargement of the right ventricle of the heart which were found, had both been undetectable by the ordinary "routine" physical exam Loki had been given earlier that year. Since he was free of any symptoms related to these changes, no treatment was necessary.

The only modification suggested was to reduce him somewhat. Loki had reached fifty pounds when he was six and, being small for a standard poodle, was more than "pleasingly plump" and actually on the verge of becoming obese. Food volume was judiciously decreased and in six months he was down to forty-five, and when he reached the age of eight, he looked great at thirty-seven pounds. He kept his trim figure and stayed within two pounds of that weight for the rest of his life. His second geriatric exam came when this handsome poodle was eight and a half. It showed a barely perceptible increase in the right ventricle enlargement, no further change in the kidney situation and complete freedom from any abnormal symptoms.

Despite having had distemper as a puppy, Loki's teeth were not stained or pitted as is often seen in other such dogs. In fact, his teeth were so good, they needed a complete dental prophylaxis treatment only twice, once when he was nine and again at eleven, with nary a single tooth needing extraction.

At his tenth year geriatric exam, the kidneys and heart were unchanged and still symptom free, but his prostate gland was slightly enlarged. This responded well to initial therapy, but there were minor flare-ups several times during the next two years. His exam at twelve showed the kidneys and heart still status quo and the prostate quite normal. But Loki's first major illness since puppyhood was just around the corner.

Four months after the exam he developed a severe kidney and prostate infection which took almost seven weeks to cure. Diane became an "expert" at giving oral medications, collecting urine specimens, and describing the contour of Loki's bowel movements (the pressure of an enlarged prostate against the rectum tends to flatten the bowel movement from top to bottom). Although Loki was a fighter when it came to being sick, it was really Diane's wonderful nursing and loving care that pulled him through this illness.

Barely recovered, Loki, one morning suddenly developed a stiff neck, arched back, weakness in all legs, and pain whenever he moved. Diane was waiting for me when I arrived at my clinic. X rays confirmed intervertebral disc disease in the neck *and* lower back. Another owner might have opted for surgical correction which, in Loki's case, would have meant less aftercare. Not Diane! "If Loki can be cured without an operation I'll do anything to make it possible." And so she did, from cleaning up the occasional bowel and urine accidents to carrying him in and out whenever necessary; and in between, giving him oral medication, administering physiotherapy, and bringing him in for reexamination and evaluation. In just over five weeks, Loki was functioning almost normally and in two months was back to his customary activities.

A small skin lump on his back was removed two months before Loki's thirteenth birthday, and we all breathed a huge sigh of relief a week later when the pathologist reported it to be a benign dermal cyst. Just one week before that birthday the dog's urine became bloody, and he strained every time he urinated. Radiographic examination revealed many very small, gravel-like calculi or "stones" in his bladder. Diane was reluctant to give her consent for the operation which was recommended, hoping she would be able to cure Loki medically as she had the intervertebral disc disease. I advised her that this was virtually impossible, but she wanted to try. Within a week, medication did clear up the symptoms, and he was freely passing normal-looking urine. Follow-up X rays over the next three months showed the calculi actually were getting smaller, and perhaps Diane was on her way to becoming a miracle worker. But this was not meant to be.

One night, when he was almost thirteen and a half, Loki began to have repeated convulsions which responded poorly to all attempts at controlling them. A chest X ray showed many small tumors throughout the lungs, making surgery impossible, despite the fact that nothing was visible on chest X rays taken only six months before. Consultation with a veterinary neurologist confirmed a rapidly growing malignancy which had spread to the brain. The prognosis was very grave, with expected survival time of only several days, or a week or two at most. Within less than one day, Loki lost control of his legs, his ability to raise his head, and almost all of his vision, in spite of intensive therapy. Because he was beginning to suffer, and nothing could be done to alleviate it, euthanasia was our recommendation and Diane's decision.

"Tinker Belle"—Chihuahua—female—
June 17, 1957, to August 30, 1974—age 17

The very first time I met Tinker Belle, she let me know that she did not particularly approve of me taking her temperature or, for that matter, of any other part of my examination. She sure was a feisty dog right from the start! But I overlooked her objections, perhaps because she was born on the same day of June as I was, and so began a long relationship.

Except for very *ir*regularly administered booster vaccinations, Tinker saw little of me until she was eight when, upon returning from North Carolina, the family homestead, her tonsils became infected. These bothered her on and off for half a year, and just as we were considering taking them out, they suddenly became normal and stayed that way. I'm convinced Tinker just decided that she wasn't going to be hospitalized and have to put up with me every day. The following winter, she started to drink a lot of water, vomit, have diarrhea, and experience difficulty in walking with her back legs. A high white blood cell count, fever, and a very tense distended abdomen, all coming as they did shortly after she finished her heat period, suggested a uterine infection. Radiographs confirmed that this was a pyometra, the uterus filled with pus being clearly visible.

I advised immediate surgery but Tony, Tinker's owner, was reluctant. His dog had never had any serious medical problems, and suddenly she now needed a major operation. He would have to talk it over with his wife who, incidentally, had never once been to my office. The next morning Tinker passed a small amount of the pus out of her vagina, and Tony and the Mrs. thought she was all better. When I still recommended surgery, explaining that there was a lot more pus where that had come from, he again said he'd have to discuss it with his wife, but he did not want me to X-ray the dog the next day. The second X ray showed no significant change in the uterus, and meanwhile Tinker was getting sicker and weaker. Finally, three days after the diagnosis had been made, and Tinker could no longer stand up, authorization for surgery was given.

The uterus was so distended, it was on the verge of rupturing. The surgery had to proceed very slowly to avoid such an event, thereby extending the duration of the operation and the anesthetic time. The liver and kidneys were visibly enlarged and swollen, confirming the damage we already knew of from the preoperative blood tests. Once the uterus, ovaries, and ligaments were removed, Tinker's breathing became less labored, and I became more hopeful. The membrane which lines the abdominal cavity as well as the subcutaneous tissue were both in such a poor state of health that extra stitches were needed when the abdominal incision was sewn closed, again prolonging anesthetic time. It was touch and go for the next five days, as Tinker would not eat, had to be fed intravenously and by stomach tube, and her body temperature remained dangerously below normal.

On the sixth day, she was once more back to herself, acting as if nothing had ever happened, eating with interest, and moving about normally. Tony took her home with instructions to keep her confined and inactive. Within two weeks she was fully recovered, had her skin stitches removed, and figured she could forget about me.

Tony was so happy to have her home and well that he started to indulge her every whim even more than before, and that included extra food. By the end of the year, he and his Mrs. had succeeded in making Tinker fatter than when she had her swollen uterus, now tipping the scales at eight and a half pounds. And so started a continuing "battle of the bulge" which was never really won until old age. When I saw Tinker two years later for a skin problem, Tony's "reducing" program had brought this Chihuahua's weight *up* to nine and a half pounds! I again explained the dangers of obesity and outlined a proper reducing program which was followed only intermittently, so it took more than two years to get her back to eight and a half.

It seemed as though that was Tinker's rock bottom weight and she could lose no more. But when she started having fainting spells at almost fifteen, due to a cardiac arrhythmia, Tony and his wife renewed their efforts, and the bulging belly was brought down to just a bit over seven pounds within one year. And there it remained. So did the arrhythmia, but with only rare fainting episodes, until midway through Tinker's sixteenth year.

Chronic congestive heart failure began to develop and was controlled fairly well for six months with specific therapy, in addition to medication for the abnormal rhythm. One night shortly before her seventeenth birthday she started crying in pain, pacing about and frequently walking backwards. Tony brought her to my clinic a little after midnight, her abdomen swollen with fluid (ascites), her tongue already turning dark. She was in acute congestive heart failure. Vigorous emergency measures to get oxygen into her lungs, remove the accumulated fluid, and support the weakening heart were only briefly helpful. Tinker Belle's heart stopped beating and could not be restarted.

We had all put up a good battle against death, and I felt professionally satisfied that nothing more could have been done. But a greater satisfaction, certainly among my most memorable ones, arrived about a week later in the mail. A half page torn from a memo pad, written on in a trembling hand, and spotted with what must have been tears, read simply, "Just a short note to thank you for the years of Pleasure you gave us with little Tinker belle. Mr. & Mrs. Antonio E."

Appendix II: What to Do in Selected Emergencies

Appendix III: Nutrient Requirements of Dogs†

Percentage or Amount per Kilogram of Food

	Type of Diet			
	Dry Basis	*Dry Type*	*Semimoist*	*Canned or Wet*
Moisture level (%)	0	10	25	75
Dry matter basis (%)	100	90	75	25
Nutrient	Requirement			
Protein %	22	20	16.5	5.5
Fat %	5.0	4.5	3.75	1.25
Linoleic acid %	1.0	0.9	0.75	0.25
Minerals				
Calcium %	1.1	1.0	0.8	0.3
Phosphorus %	0.9	0.8	0.7	0.22
Potassium %	0.6	0.5	0.45	0.2
Sodium chloride %	1.1	1.0	0.8	0.3
Magnesium %	0.040	0.036	0.030	0.010
Iron mg	60	54	45	15
Copper mg	7.3	6.5	5.5	1.8
Manganese mg	5.0	4.5	3.8	1.2
Zinc mg	50	45	38	12
Iodine mg	1.54	1.39	1.16	0.39
Selenium mg	0.11	0.10	0.08	0.03
Vitamins				
Vitamin A IU	5000	4500	3750	1250
Vitamin D IU	500	450	375	125
Vitamin E IU	50	45	37.5	12.5
Thiamin mg	1.00	0.90	0.75	0.25
Riboflavin mg	2.2	2.0	1.6	0.5
Pantothenic acid mg	10.0	9.0	7.5	2.5
Niacin mg	11.4	10.3	8.6	2.8
Pyridoxine mg	1.0	0.9	0.75	0.25
Folic acid mg	0.18	0.16	0.14	0.04
Biotin mg	0.10	0.09	0.075	0.025
Vitamin B_{12} mg	0.022	0.020	0.017	0.006
Choline mg	1200	1100	900	300

† % = percentage of food by weight; gm = grams; mg = milligrams; IU = international units; μg = micrograms.

Per Kilogram of Body Weight per Day

Nutrient	*Units*	*Adult Maintenance*
Protein	gm	4.8
Fat	gm	1.1
Linoleic acid	gm	0.22
Minerals		
Calcium	mg	242
Phosphorus	mg	198
Potassium	mg	132
Sodium chloride	mg	242
Magnesium	mg	8.8
Iron	mg	1.32
Copper	mg	0.16
Manganese	mg	0.11
Zinc	mg	1.1
Iodine	mg	0.034
Selenium	μg	2.42
Vitamins		
Vitamin A	IU	110
Vitamin D	IU	11
Vitamin E	IU	1.1
Thiamin	μg	22
Riboflavin	μg	48
Pantothenic acid	μg	220
Niacin	μg	250
Pyridoxine	μg	22
Folic acid	μg	4.0
Biotin	μg	2.2
Vitamin B_{12}	μg	0.5
Choline	mg	26

Adapted from *Nutrient Requirements of Dogs* (ISBN 0-309-02315-7), Committee on Animal Nutrition, National Research Council, National Academy of Sciences, Washington, D.C., 1974.

Appendix IV: Tables

Normal Physiological Values for Dogs

Body temperature	100°–102.2°F (37.8°–39°C)
Pulse (heart rate)	70–160 beats per minute
Respiration rate	10–30 per minute
Red blood cells	5.5–8.5 million per cubic millimeter
White blood cells	6000–17000 per cubic millimeter
Hemoglobin	12–17 grams per 100 milliliters
Red blood cell life span	100–120 days

Canine Body Temperature Equivalents in °F and °C

Fahrenheit to Celsius	
94	34.4
95	35.0
96	35.6
97	36.1
98	36.7
99	37.2
100	37.8
101	38.3
102	38.9
103	39.4
104	40.0
105	40.6
106	41.1
107	41.7
108	42.2

Celsius to Fahrenheit	
34	93.2
35	95.0
36	96.8
37	98.6
38	100.4
39	102.2
40	104.0
41	105.8
42	107.6

Conversion Factors

Fahrenheit to Celsius (centigrade)	degrees F − 32 × 5/9
Celsius to Fahrenheit	degrees C × 9/5 + 32
Pounds to grams (approximate)	× 454
Grams to pounds (approximate)	× 0.0022
Pounds to kilograms (approximate)	× 2.2
Kilograms to pounds (approximate)	× 0.454

Weight Equivalents

1 pound = 453.6 grams = 0.4536 kilograms = 16 ounces
1 ounce = 28.35 grams
1 kilogram = 1000 grams = 2.2046 pounds
1 gram = 1000 milligrams
1 milligram = 1000 micrograms

Glossary

Adrenal gland—located adjacent to, and just in front of, each kidney, it secretes several types of steroid and other hormones.

Amino acid—the primary building block of protein. Of the many types known, at least nine are essential for the maintenance of good health in the dog.

Anemia—less than the normal number of red blood cells, or amount of hemoglobin.

Arrhythmia—any alteration in the normal rhythm of the heart beat.

Arthrodese—to obliterate and fuse a joint in the skeleton by surgical procedure.

Ascites—the accumulation of fluid in the abdominal cavity.

Atrium (pl. atria)—the upper chamber(s) of the heart.

Atrophy—a shrinking or wasting away.

Auscultation—listening to sounds inside the body. Can be done with the ear alone or more often with a stethoscope.

Balanoposthitis—an inflammation of the prepuce or sheath covering the penis.

Benign—not malignant.
Brachycephalic—having a short, wide head with "pushed in" face, e.g., pug, pekingese, boxer, English bulldog.
Bronchiole—a small tubular branching of the larger bronchi.
Bronchus (pl. bronchi)—the large main tubular air passage(s) connecting the trachea with the lungs.

Calculus—the hard mineral tartar deposited on the surface of a tooth.
Carcinogenic—the capability of a given substance to produce cancer.
Cataract—an opacity of the lens of the eye.
Cecum—a blind end intestinal pouch located where the small and large intestines join.
Chemotherapy—the treatment of disorders with various chemicals.
Colitis—an inflammation of the colon, or large intestine.
Congenital—present at the time of birth but not necessarily hereditary.
Conjunctiva—the pink membrane which lines the eyelids and covers the adjacent areas of the eyeball.
Cornea—the clear "window" which forms the front of the eyeball.
Corticosteroid—any of several hormones produced by the adrenal glands.
Cryosurgery—destroying and removing tissue by controlled freezing.

Debilitating—producing weakness and loss of strength.
Definitive diagnosis—the specific cause of a disorder determined with great certainty.
Dermatitis—an inflammation of the skin.
Diabetes insipidus—a metabolic disease of the pituitary gland which reduces the kidneys' ability to resorb water, resulting in very large amounts of urine.
Diabetes mellitus—a metabolic disease of the pancreas resulting in a high blood sugar level, sugar in the urine, and large amounts of urine.
Differential diagnosis—the consideration and comparison of two

or more possible different disorders in order to arrive at the one definitive diagnosis.

Digitalis—one of a group of drugs used to strengthen the contractile force of the heart and slow its rate of contraction.

Diuretic—a drug which increases the production of urine.

Embolism—the sudden mechanical obstruction of an artery, usually by a blood clot formed elsewhere in the body.

Endemic—continually present in a given area; as endemic disease.

Endocrine organ—an organ which produces substances (hormones) that are secreted directly into the blood and cause a response in other organs.

Enucleation—the removal of an organ or structure *in toto;* "peeling out."

Enzyme—a protein compound which speeds up, or otherwise enhances, specific chemical processes in the body.

Epithelium—the covering of the outside of the body as well as that of its inner surfaces.

Familial—having a tendency to affect various members of a family.

Flatulence—the excessive accumulation of gas in the intestines.

Gingiva—the gums of the mouth.

Glaucoma—increased pressure of the fluid within the eyeball which can lead to blindness.

Hock joint—the first joint up from the toes, in the hind leg, which points toward the rear of the dog. Equivalent to the human heel, in a healthy dog it does not touch the ground during walking.

Hyperglycemia—an abnormally high level of glucose (sugar) in the blood.

Hyperplasia—an increase in the *number* of otherwise normal cells.

Hypertrophy—an increase in the *size* of otherwise normal cells.

Hypoglycemia—an abnormally low level of glucose (sugar) in the blood.

Hypothalamus—that part of the brain which forms its underside and includes the pituitary gland and the crossing of the optic nerves.

Idiopathic—a way of saying that the specific cause of an illness is unknown.

Idiosyncrasy—a unique individual peculiarity or susceptibility.

Insuloma—a tumor of the insulin secreting cells of the pancreas.

Keratoconjunctivitis sicca—an inflammation and drying out of the cornea and conjunctiva of the eye caused by insufficient tear secretion.

Ketoacidosis—a serious life-threatening complication of untreated diabetes mellitus.

Lacrimal gland—the tear gland of the eye.

Leptospirosis—a disease of the urinary system in dogs.

Malignant—highly active with a tendency to get worse; cancerous.

Metabolism—the total of all bodily processes by which living tissue and energy are produced from ingested food, water, and oxygen.

Metastasis—the spread of disease from one organ, or part of the body, to a distant one. Used most often when referring to tumors.

Mitral valve—the valve separating the upper and lower chambers on the left side of the heart.

Musculoskeletal—relating to the skeleton and muscles.

Mutation—a sudden permanent new characteristic in an offspring which is different from that in its parents.

Nebulization—changing a liquid into a fine spray, such as with an atomizer.

Nuclear sclerosis—a normal thickening and hardening of the fibers in the center of the lens of the eye.

Nocturia—increased urination during the night.

Optic nerve—transmits visual impulses from the eye to the brain.

Ovariohysterectomy—the surgical removal of the ovaries and uterus; spay.

Palliative—tending to give temporary relief, but not to cure.
Palpation—the examination of the body by feeling with the fingers and hands.
Paraplegia—paralysis of the hind legs and rear parts of the body.
Patella—the knee cap.
Pathognomonic—a sign or symptoms so specifically characteristic of a disease that a definitive diagnosis can be made from it alone.
Percussion—the striking of a body part in order to diagnose the health of the underlying structures from the sound produced.
Periodontal—the area immediately surrounding a tooth.
pH—the symbol used to indicate the degree of alkalinity or acidity. pH 7 is neutral; higher than 7 is alkaline; and less than 7 is acid.
Physiotherapy—the treatment of illness by physical, as opposed to medical, means, e.g., massage.
Pituitary gland—a small gland situated on the underside of the brain which secretes many different hormones.
Plaque—the soft deposits on the surface of a tooth in which bacteria and minerals accumulate.
Pleural effusion—the presence of fluid in the small spaces between the lungs and the chest wall.
Prepuce—the foreskin of the penis.
Prognosis—the prediction of the probable course and outcome of a disease.
Prophylaxis—preventive treatment.
Prosthetic—the replacement of a natural body part by an artificial one.
Provisional diagnosis—a tentative or temporary determination to be used until further testing or examination yields a definitive diagnosis.
Pseudocyesis—a false pregnancy.
Pulmonary edema—the presence of fluid in the air cells and tissues of the lungs.
Pyometra—the accumulation of pus inside the uterus.

Radiation therapy—the treatment of illness with X rays, radium or other radioactive materials.
Radiograph—a picture made by means of radioactivity which shows the structures within the body; an x-ray picture.

Scale (teeth)—to scrape tartar from the surfaces of the teeth.
Sclera—the white portion of the eyeball.
Senility—old age accompanied by mental and physical infirmity.
Spay—to perform an ovariohysterectomy.
Stifle joint—the first joint down from the hip, in the hind leg, which points toward the front of the dog. It is equivalent to the human knee.
Subcutaneously—just beneath the skin.
Symmetrical—occurring equally on both sides of a middle line; usually, but not always, a mirror image.
Syndrome—a group of signs or symptoms occurring together which may or may not cause a specific disorder or illness.

Toxic (toxin)—poisonous (a poison).
Tricuspid valve—the valve separating the upper and lower chambers on the right side of the heart.

Uremia—a toxic state caused by the presence in the blood of abnormally high levels of urea and other waste products of metabolism normally excreted by the kidneys into the urine.

Ventricle(s)—the lower chamber(s) of the heart.

Index